The Essential Herbal for Natural Health

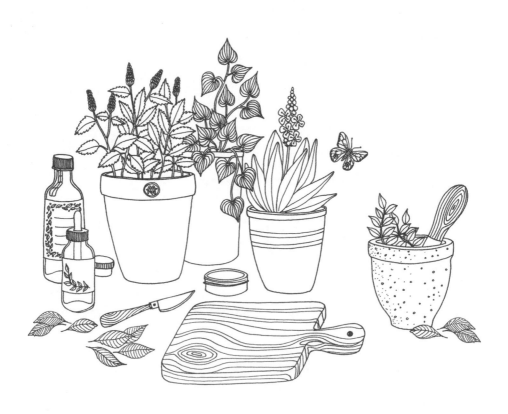

THE ESSENTIAL HERBAL FOR NATURAL HEALTH

*How to Transform Easy-to-Find
Herbs into Healing Remedies
for the Whole Family*

Holly Bellebuono

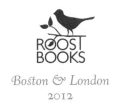

ROOST
BOOKS

Boston & London
2012

Roost Books
An imprint of Shambhala Publications, Inc.
Horticultural Hall
300 Massachusetts Avenue
Boston, Massachusetts 02115
roostbooks.com

9 8 7 6 5 4 3 2 1

First Edition
Printed in the United States of America

♾ This edition is printed on acid-free paper that meets the American National Standards Institute Z39.48 Standard.
♻ Shambhala Publications makes every effort to print on recycled paper. For more information please visit www.shambhala.com.

Distributed in the United States by Random House, Inc., and in Canada by Random House of Canada Ltd

Dedication

To Mom and Dad, for supporting and inspiring me.
To Rocco, for being a wonderful husband and father.
To Gabriel and Madia, for the joy
you've both brought into my life.

May this book inspire many creative endeavors.

Contents

Fourteen years ago, I walked across the long bridge over the Watauga River in Sugar Grove, North Carolina. The rural valley was dotted with farm-houses and barns, and wildflowers blanketed the riverbank. I turned right at the abandoned yet structurally sound Farthing farmhouse and entered what appeared to be a last remnant of old-growth hemlocks, towering and quiet. Rhododendron grew beneath them like little plump balls of green, and here and there a sheep or a cow lay at the foot of a massive hemlock trunk. Ahead of me, on the lower slope of the mountain, sat a little 1950s brick ranch and beyond that the original farmhouse for this holler (valley), abandoned and used for storage. On the brick ranch's doorstep, a woman appeared—stocky, in her fifties or sixties, and sensibly dressed. I had al-ready discovered that everything about Georgia Gillis was very sensible: her dress, her collection of historical artifacts and photographs from the region, even her approach to livestock and farming—she had turned part of the valley she inherited into a Christmas tree farm.

"Going out again today?" she asked, grinning.

"Yes ma'am," I replied.

Georgia nodded and led me past the long-abandoned farmhouse farther up the hill, explaining again that this had been her family's homestead and that she and all her siblings had grown up here. I peeked in the windows as we walked past. An old iron water pump still presided over the enamel sink; wooden crates sat tucked under old sash windows.

For several years, I'd spent every spare moment following old-timers into the deep blue forests of southern Appalachia, and since I'd moved into this beautiful valley and, by chance, had met this guardian lady of the mountainside, I'd shown up regularly on Georgia's front porch to ask if she was heading up into the hills that day. Invariably she was, and I would have the good fortune to tag along and learn some of her folk-healing wisdom.

Georgia raised Scottish Highland cattle, giant soft-brown creatures that intimidated me with their long curved horns and shaggy coats, but what they really wanted was to be petted. She opened the gate and pushed a massive cow away by its soft nose. "Go on, now," she ordered. The cow pestered her for attention, and she swatted at it, gently but firmly, with a rolled-up newspaper. The massive horned cow ambled away and left us to walk over creeks dotted with wild mint and into the cool of high-altitude beech forests.

In her calm, no-nonsense voice, Georgia taught me many of the wild botanicals she and her ancestors had relied on as medicine for generations. It was old hat for her. Normal. Nothing to be aroused by. But to me, the fact that wildflowers and weeds could not only be eaten but could heal was novel. I discovered crimson-colored wake-robin (trillium), creamy white bloodroot, and one that baffled me before I realized Georgia's "bum-gilly" referred to the greasy balm of Gilead buds of the tulip poplar tree. Plantain, the curse of many a front yard, was one of Georgia's favorites, and she showed me how to chew the leaf and apply it to a bee sting for instant relief.

Other kind mountain folks generously gave of their time, and over the course of a couple of years, I wandered through ancient groves of 500-year-old cherry trees, mountain trails sprinkled with blue larkspur, and protected forests nurturing gorgeous wild orchids. I basked in the delicious pleasures of crisp Solomon's seal root pulled from the earth, chickweed straight from a cold spring, dandelion, red clover, wild stinging nettles, fragrant hemlock tips, and juicy (though inedible) poke root.

Of course, I immediately wanted to make things with them. As someone who likes to make things with my hands, my driving desire was to enjoy the riches of Mother Nature through the alluring jewel boxes of glass bottles, jars, tincture dispensers, and cream pots. I've always been handy and have been known to sew clothes, quilt, can and preserve all manner of vegetables and fruits, set yogurt, weave pine needle basketry, carve soapstone, make hummus and sauces, spin pottery, decoupage plates—bringing varying degrees of talent to each endeavor. I believe it's a gift of my Appalachian heritage; mountain folk generally hailed from Scotland and Ireland and were famously independent and reclusive. The Scotch-Irish colonizers of western North Carolina made nearly everything they needed and were renowned for their craftiness, inventiveness, and creativity.

There is Scotch-Irish blood in me along with German and some Native American. These cultures value the handcraft arts and the ability to make from nature the tools and treasures of sustenance and fortitude. We can thank our foremothers and forefathers for the toys, foods, fibers, paints, clothing, structures, medicines, and other valuables they fashioned from the giving plants of the field and forest. Today this is a science called ethno-botany. Then, it was a way of life.

During my first years as an herbalist, after Georgia left me on my own to chop and mix and pound green plants to my heart's content, I experimented with making herbal concoctions from the common weeds I found in every meadow. My counters groaned under the weight of countless glass mason jars of dandelion root vinegar; comfrey ointment; violet elixir; and aromatic, herb-based bug repellent. My medicine cabinet held bottles of every imaginable size and shape, but after a season the sticky-note labels would fall off, and I would be left wondering what was inside each bottle of strong-smelling, colorful liquid. (This was a useful lesson in proper labeling.) My dog became the benefactor of numerous plantain, peppermint, calendula, rosemary, or Saint-John's-wort oil applications; every paw received a rubbing, and any sign of a scratch or cut was promptly smeared.

Since then, I've refined my techniques, learned more about methodology, and been introduced to countless more plants and their intricacies. I've traveled throughout the Appalachian mountains and to England, Scotland, Ireland, Holland, the Pacific Northwest, and Hawaii in search of the communities and individuals who've awakened their passion for plants to fashion a way of life. I've been blessed to receive teachings by master healers such as Rocio Alarcon of Ecuador and Zapotecan midwife Doña Enriqueta Contreras, who shared with me some of their beautiful bathing therapies using floral waters and rose petals. I've pulled (and tasted) weeds in gardens from Fairview, North Carolina, to the Findhorn Foundation community on Scotland's North Sea coast. My formulas reflect not only a basic earned knowledge of pharmacology and chemistry but also a honed sense of intuition, as I've learned from each batch and monitored the herbs' effects on my own body and on those of willing friends and colleagues. Today I make and sell more than seventy original formulas through my business, Vineyard Herbs Teas & Apothecary, all of which are a result of learning from others, listening to the plants, and being open to experimentation and "outer" guidance.

The simple yet effective recipes in this book are the result of centuries of herbalists sharing collective wisdom, for which I am profoundly grateful, and of my twenty years of general trial and error and fifteen years of professional formulation. Through this book, I hope to contribute something useful to our wonderful heritage of herbal knowledge. As you enter the world of herbalism, above all, enjoy the process, love the plants, and share what you learn.

Acknowledgments

Many hands and hearts have contributed to my growing knowledge of herbal medicine and to this book.

Many heartfelt thanks go to all my dear girlfriends who, for years, have supported my pursuit of herbal knowledge and my career: Sara Figlow, Mary Ambulos, Isabel Proffitt, Sandra Guerrero, Linda Hilyard, and Lisa Benson. Much love and appreciation to Gini Crowder-Marshall, Pat Reinhardt, Heather Thurber, Kim Klaren, Susan Marbell, and Elizabeth Stratton.

Special thanks go to my wonderful sister, Leslie Roberts, who is the best girlfriend of them all, and to Laurisa Rich, who has enthusiastically apprenticed with me for years. A cosmic thank-you and walk by the river to Janice Aquaviva, who mentored me early on and taught me to listen to intuition. And I am very grateful to Joanne Brownstein and Jennifer Urban-Brown for their tirelessly creative and nurturing work toward the production of this book.

I would especially like to acknowledge the plants: the herbs, flowers, and trees with their greenery, fresh air, and electric energy. Many thanks go to the forests of Appalachia and the meadows of Martha's Vineyard.

Most of all, I am grateful to my husband and best friend, Rocco, who has supported all my endeavors and encouraged me to embrace my path as a healer, an herbalist, and a writer.

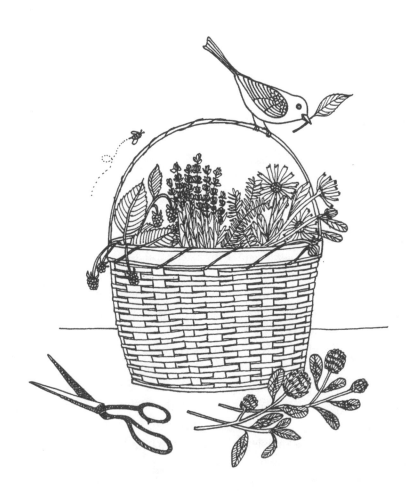

Part One

THE HERBS

My love affair with nature is so deep that I am not satisfied with being a mere onlooker, or nature tourist. I crave a more real and meaningful relationship. The spicy teas and tasty delicacies I prepare from wild ingredients are the bread and wine in which I have communion and fellowship with nature, and with the Author of that nature.

—Euell Gibbons

Chapter One

INTRODUCING
HERBS AND HERBALISM

What is herbal medicine? In general, an *herb* is a flower, shrub, tree, or even seaweed that has been cultivated or harvested for use in culinary or medicinal applications. Long before herbs were the backbone of a multi-million-dollar-a-year industry in the United States, they were the simple, unassuming yet essential mainstay of health for most of the world's population. They didn't paste labels on themselves or package themselves in fancy containers. Instead, herbs simply grew and healed. Countless families learned how to use herbs from their parents and grandparents, and they later passed this same knowledge down to their children.

This heritage has blessed us today with an understanding of hundreds of safe, readily available healing herbs. While a handful of these have gone on to shine as stars in complicated pharmaceutical formulas and secure approval by several countries' governments, most herbs are content to be considered backyard weeds. And these little weeds can be our best resource for getting and staying healthy! So much of our plant heritage teaches us to use what is plentiful, grows nearby, and is proven safe. Such are herbs—either garden grown or "wildcrafted."

Wildcrafted means plants that are identified growing in their natural habitat and then harvested on the spot for use in herbal medicines. The art of identifying and wildcrafting herbs was nearly lost during the industrial era—and certainly rejected during the space age—but, thankfully, it is making a comeback. People are more and more interested in learning what the heck those green plants are that they see growing in the meadows, fields, and woodlands around them and, even more, what the heck they can do with those plants. They're useful? Yes!

Harvesting your own plants, whether they are grown in a greenhouse or garden or wildcrafted from a nearby field, is a very satisfying endeavor and one I happily commend if you want to make your own medicines or even cook in your kitchen. Getting familiar with oregano, lemon balm, and sage from the garden, or yarrow, elder, and red clover from the field, is well worth the effort and will reward you with many delicious and nutritious meals and remedies.

Of the many reasons you'll find satisfaction in this process (including being in the fresh air, learning a new skill, and heightening your awareness of the natural world), surely the most enticing is the fact that making natural herbal remedies will take you down the path toward safe, easy, and healthy self-sufficiency. You need not be dependent on the pharmaceutical industry or the medical establishment—although balance is very healthy; I, for one, am grateful for the benefits that modern medicine offers for emergency care, diagnosis, and the treatment of trauma, broken bones, and intense bacterial and viral infections. However, I value the centuries of healing gained from herbal medicine for treating common or chronic disorders of the mind and body, generally without dangerous complications, side effects, or addictions.

USING FRESH HERBS

When making medicines (with the exception of infusions, powders, and suppositories), fresh herbs are almost always preferable to dried. Fresh herbs still retain a certain "green living energy" that the body can use to heal, and they possess much of the essential oil content that can be lost during drying.

Fresh herbs can be prepared and used in simple ways; water-based methods include teas and infusions (though dried herbs work best here), decoctions, syrups, compresses, poultices, and hydrosols. These have a short shelf life and should be used quickly, sometimes within minutes of making the remedy. Fresh herbs are choice ingredients in tinctures, including those with alcohol, glycerin, and vinegar bases, which have a longer shelf life than water-based preparations and are portable. Fresh herbs are also better than dried for making oils and salves, though they should be slightly wilted before using. (Details on all of these types of remedies are described in chapter 4: Medicine-Making Methods.)

I prefer fresh herbs because I harvest many plants myself, and the freshest plant is the most potent plant energetically. By all means, enjoy fresh plants frequently—inhale, touch, and nibble. Establishing relationships with fresh, live plants is invaluable and, in my opinion, the first step toward any healing.

USING DRIED HERBS

Dried plants offer certain benefits as well: they can be purchased from other locations around the world, giving us the fantastic opportunity to experience a wide range of botanical remedies and experiment with healing methods from different cultures. Dried plants work best in powders and capsules, since they can be ground and mixed with arrowroot for body powder or measured into gelatin capsules for "pill-like" remedies. They are also preferable in infusions.

Dried plants, since they have released their water content, require less liquid in recipes than fresh plants do. When substituting dried plant material for fresh, follow this guideline:

Fresh plants: full measure in recipe
Dried plants: one-third measure in recipe

In other words, if a recipe calls for 3 teaspoons of fresh herbs, you may substitute 1 teaspoon of dried herbs.

Drying Herbs

I have found several methods to dry freshly harvested herbs, depending on the climate and weather conditions.

In damp or cold climates, spread the herbs in a single layer on a wire rack or baking sheet. Place them in an electric, gas, or solar oven on very low heat of about 100° F for several hours until crisp. Store them in a zip-lock bag or (even better) a glass jar with a tight-fitting lid.

In dry or warm climates, spread the herbs in a single layer on a large screen. I've had great luck with old door-size screens. Balance the screen on top of two sawhorses or similar supports in the shade, and let the herbs dry until they are crisp. Store them as already described.

I've also successfully dried many stems, stalks, leafy greens (such as sage and mint), and flowers by hanging them in bunches from the rafters in a breezy attic. The warmth and circulating air dries them, while the darkness keeps the colors vibrant. If you wish to collect the seeds from your dried herbs, bunch the herbs together with string and hang them upside down *inside* a large paper bag. They will dry and release their seeds into the bag, so you can collect them easily.

CHOOSING FRESH OR DRIED HERBS

When should you use fresh and when dried? As with any questions that arise during medicine making, I recommend listening to the voice of intuition as a guide to harvesting, creating, and using herbal medicines. Listen to the plants. Stand still in the forest or field and let what will come, come. Intuition's guidance is as valuable as any class you can take. Blended with a little science and a pinch of research, reflection and inner guidance are powerful teachers.

Chapter Two

THE ESSENTIAL HERBS

While there are countless useful herbs in the world, the recipes in this book focus on thirteen primary herbs—a baker's dozen, if you will—that can form the cornerstone of a foray into herbal medicine making. I find myself coming back to these particular herbs time and again, and most of my formulas include one or more of them.

The Essential Herbs, as I refer to them, are those that serve multiple purposes. They give the most bang for the buck, and the time you spend learning about them will reward you with a wide range of effective remedies. I've established the following criteria for selecting these particular herbs:

- They are easy to find and identify (either in cultivation or in the wild).
- They are common (many are "weeds").
- None of them is on any endangered, threatened, or at-risk list.
- They are versatile and can be used to treat a variety of ailments.
- They are established, effective herbs that have been used for centuries.

- They are safe.
- It is easy to make medicines and foods with them.

These criteria ensure that the Essential Herbs will provide pleasurable herbal crafting, especially for the beginning herbalist. By incorporating them into your herbal repertoire, these formulas will give you a strong foundation in making herbal medicines, or—if you're already familiar with botanical healing—they will give you a basis for branching off in more exotic directions using solid, proven recipes.

The Essential Herbs are as follows:

Calendula
Dandelion
Elder
Ginger
Lavender
Lemon balm
Mint
Nettle
Plantain
Raspberry
Red clover
Rose
Yarrow

Almost all of them can be grown successfully in the home garden, even in pots on a windowsill. The few that aren't generally cultivated can be found easily; you can harvest elder in many meadows or pastures, and ginger is readily available at the grocery store.

While these herbs form the foundation to the recipes in the following chapters, I've included other herbs as well. Used in conjunction with the basic herbs, they enhance the desired effects of a remedy or act as a "delivery vehicle" to refine the effects in the body. The recipes are presented as simply as possible while offering a diverse range of remedies especially for the beginner.

CALENDULA
Calendula officinalis

Calendula, a cousin of the marigold, is so named because it stays colorful and vivid throughout the calendar year, lasting throughout the changing seasons. It can easily be grown in a garden or even on a windowsill. It is at once sunshiny and proper, growing in neat clumps without spreading or taking over. The reddish orange and yellow flower heads break off easily, and I always cut off the pouch with the black and white filaments, using only the deeply colored petals in my oils. This gives a vibrant color and strong potency to salves. Fresh petals are best; dried petals result in a drab color and shorter shelf life.

Calendula is a most effective emollient to soothe the skin. Oil made from the crushed flowers of this plant leave skin feeling supple and soft. Prized for its ability to heal eczema and psoriasis, calendula addresses stubborn skin conditions that leave scars and blisters on the face, elbows, hands, and fingers. Apply a nourishing and strengthening calendula oil or salve to any place that is dry, calloused, bruised, stretched, or sore, and watch the healing begin. Calendula oil makes a great gift for new mothers to soothe sore nipples during breast-feeding. Consider this lovely plant a doula to keep with you before and after delivery for soothing the womb, the nipples, postpartum tears, and even your baby's fragile new skin.

Calendula is a proven and powerful antimicrobial and germ-fighter that can be used to treat wounds. You can combine it with marshmallow or lavender in a basic oil such as sweet almond or olive to make a burn cream or a cream to nourish new skin tissues. Calendula can also be used as a tincture to kill internal and external parasites, eradicate bacterial infections, or counteract a particularly bad case of sepsis.

 You'll find calendula recipes and formulas in the following chapters:

Chapter 5. For the Expectant and New Mother
Herby Sitz Bath

Chapter 6. For Infant and Child
Baby Scalp Rinse
Yeast Rinse
Baby's Calendula Thrush Rinse
Calendula Beeswax Salve
Baby Massage Oil

Chapter 7. Especially for Women
Love Your Lymph System Tea
Calendula Suppository

Chapter 11. Healing Wounds
Rosemary's Blessing First Aid Ointment

Chapter 13. Tummy Health
Bitters Tincture

Chapter 15. Cleansing and Detox
Urinary Tract Infection Tea
Summer Cleansing Infusion
Alterative Internal Tincture for Eczema
Alterative Lotion for Eczema and Psoriasis
Easy Calendula-Beeswax Salve

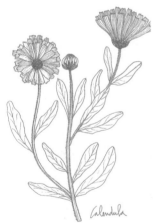

Calendula

Chapter 17. Beauty, Skin, and Body Care
Cooling Acne Wash
Calendula Facial Astringent
Herbal Lemon Hair Rinse for Light Hair

DANDELION
Taraxacum officinale

Unjustly called a pernicious weed, dandelion is one of the true great healing herbs. It's that persistent friend who won't leave you alone, showing
up in every crack in the pavement and behind every shed. In fact, its stubborn tenacity is why you need dandelion, because with regular use of this
mineral-rich herb, you'll feel brighter, stronger, lighter, and shinier.

Usually seen as a ground-level plant, this lovely herb can grow
nearly eighteen inches tall if it is in rich, shady soil and left undisturbed.
Dandelions are easily recognizable, with their deeply serrated leaves, tall
flower stalks, and bright yellow flowers that turn to wind-wispy white
seed heads—often used by children blowing on the seeds to make a wish.
(And who's to say it doesn't work?)

Its leaves are diuretic, earning it the name *piss en lit*, meaning "wet the
bed," in France. They rid the body of excess sodium but naturally replace
valuable potassium, and they are high in vitamin A. They also make superb
salad greens.

The roots are easy to harvest—they pull up in one big taproot with
lots of small roots clinging to the clump. These roots, sometimes tan or
light orange in color, are high in iron and contain liver-strengthening com-
pounds. For these reasons, dandelion root is prized as a blood-cleansing and
blood-building herb and as a liver tonic.

The easiest and most effective ways to use dandelion are to steep the fresh
roots in vinegar (see "Making a Vinegar Tincture" in chapter 4: Medicine-

Making Methods) and to enjoy the leaves fresh in foods, such as salads and sauces, and even as a pizza topping. The bitter principle present in the leaves is a wonderful digestive aid and, together with its diuretic properties, is useful in treating many conditions, including breast tenderness, premenstrual syndrome (PMS), anemia, weight gain, water retention, high blood pressure, bladder and urinary problems, cysts, gall bladder problems, and even mild pain.

 You'll find recipes and formulas using dandelion in the following chapters:

Chapter 5. For the Expectant and New Mother
Mother's Meadow Tea

Chapter 6. For Infant and Child
Candida Tincture for Nursing Mothers

Chapter 7. Especially for Women
Moon Time Vinegar Tincture
Iron-Rich Salad Dressing
Delicious Mineral Decoction
Delicious Mineral Infusion
Wild Yam PMS Jam
Lovely Hormone Tea

Chapter 9. Everyday Tonics for Vitality
Everyday Tonic for Vitality and Vigor

Chapter 12. Happy Heart
Hearty Bitters

Chapter 13. Tummy Health
Digestive Aid/Gas Relief Tincture
Bitters Tincture

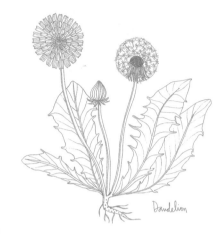

Dandelion

ELDER
Sambucus nigra, S. canadensis

The beautiful shrub elder is high on my list of most useful plants—and for good reason. Of the hundreds of beneficial plants available, I turn to it time and again during cold and flu season. Elder is renowned for its immune-strengthening abilities and its capacity to give a measure of protection against bacterial and viral infections.

I've been enamored with elder for years and have come to know her as a magician. She is a tree whose spirit seems to bend itself in many directions at once, which begins to explain the many enchanting myths about the elusive elder that have survived the centuries. Many cultures developed the concept of a woman's spirit residing in a tree, particularly in the elder. It was believed by the people of ancient Europe, Ireland, and Scotland to harbor the spirit of a strong and powerful woman who demanded a sacrifice in exchange for using parts of the tree. Ancient herbalists brought offerings to the "Elder Woman" in return for the privilege of harvesting her berries and flowers, but I believe that instead of offerings or sacrifices, the best way to honor this tree is to share your knowledge of her with others. Every part of the elder is useful: the berries, root, flowers, leaves, and even the bark and twigs that were once fashioned into small flutes.

Elder trees grow all along the eastern seaboard, but be careful you don't confuse them with the crampbark, or *Viburnum opulus*, that bloom at the same time. Elder flowers are a creamy color and blossom in the late spring and early summer here on Martha's Vineyard. *Viburnum* flowers look similar to elder but are much more compact than the loose elder blossoms, and you'll see a marked difference in the leaves too. An elder tree has long, pointy leaves, while a *Viburnum*'s are rounded and squat.

Elder flowers are known for lowering fever, especially in children. They also make a lovely, light-colored syrup. Herbalists use both elder-flower syrup and tincture to treat the common cold, influenza, upper respiratory congestion, hay fever, and sinusitis.

The berries are profuse in autumn and easy to gather; my children love to help me, and afterward, our hands are a deep, rich purple. The berries grow in clumps and can be snipped off (after requesting permission from the Elder Woman!) and then dried, frozen, or cooked (they're not good eaten raw). Because they have the same medicinal value as the flowers, they are frequently tinctured or made into a medicinal syrup. The tasty berries also make a wonderful cordial or liqueur.

You'll quickly realize your endeavors in making herbal medicines are fully satisfied by working with the lovely elder tree.

 You'll find elderberry and elder flower recipes and formulas in the following chapters:

Chapter 5. For the Expectant and New Mother
Happy Sun Tea
Elder Flower Hydrosol Spritzer
Nipple Nurse Salve

Chapter 6. For Infant and Child
Baby Scalp Rinse
Elder Flower Tincture
Children's Flu Syrup
Baby Massage Oil

Chapter 7. Especially for Women
Nipple Moisturizing Oil

Chapter 8. Especially for Men
Stress-Less Tonic Tea

Chapter 9. Everyday Tonics for Vitality
Everyday Immune Tonic
Energy Elixir

Chapter 10. Sniffles, Colds, and Viruses
Wet Cough Tea
Elderberry-Currant Honey
West Chop Winter Tea for Colds and Flu
Elderberry-Ginger Syrup for Colds and Flu
Children's Fever Friend
Herbalists' Sniffle Friend

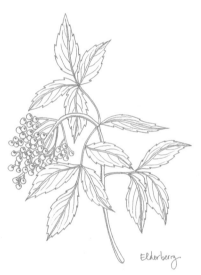

Elderberry

GINGER
Zingiber officinale

We commonly find ginger in the refrigerated aisle of the supermarket, and few of us witness it growing in its native tropical habitats, though I was lucky enough to meet it at the Waimea Arboretum and Botanical Garden on Oahu. Ginger is one of those gorgeous tropical plants that constantly renews its passport, because it falls in love with every part of the world it visits; its fiery and exotic root is on the shelf of almost every market in the world and has been a top commodity for centuries.

Beautiful with its scarlet flowers and long, slender, glossy leaves, ginger is most commonly known for its knotty root, which is thick and juicy with light tan skin. You can grow ginger in a hothouse or simply purchase it fresh, dried, or candied. Fresh root is called for in most recipes in this book, though dried root is also acceptable.

Ginger is a circulatory stimulant that warms the blood, and it is also a diaphoretic, encouraging perspiration to reduce high fevers. The old wives of Europe relied on this exotic rhizome on cold days with a cup of honey-sweetened hot tea, and they brewed it in their hearths with elderberry or mint to relieve morning and motion sickness. Today, many women use ginger for the cramps and nausea associated with PMS and pregnancy.

Externally, a poultice of shredded boiled ginger or a strong ginger tea compress can ease rheumatism and arthritis.

 You'll find ginger recipes and formulas in the following chapters:

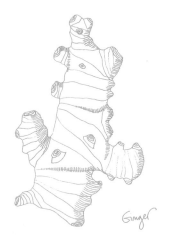

Chapter 5. For the Expectant and New Mother
Wild Yam Infusion
Fennel-Ginger Tea
Good Morning Bites

Chapter 6. For Infant and Child
Children's Digestive Glycerite

Chapter 7. Especially for Women
Love Your Lymph System Tea

Chapter 8. Especially for Men
"Get to the Root of the Problem" Prostate Tonic
Chilmark Chai
Deep Forest Massage Oil
Foot Soak

Ginger

LAVENDER
Lavandula officinalis, L. angustifolia

A cultivated herb, lavender has enjoyed a love affair with humanity since ancient times. Hailed as a toiletry herb, it is a common ingredient in bath salts, perfume, and soaps—indeed, its name comes from the Latin *lavare*, meaning "to wash." Lavender has long been associated with water, infusing soaps and oils with the renewing and sensual scent of summer.

Smell-good plants—especially those whose blossoms can be infused in precious oils—earned the name *nard* in the Bible, and the "spikenard" in the Song of Solomon may be lavender. Nicholas Culpeper, in 1653, noted that oil of lavender is "usually called oil of spike," which refers to the tall-stemmed flower. The herb grows in a loose mound with hundreds of purple-tipped flower stems reaching upward, clothed by silvery gray, narrow leaves; these leaves also impart a lovely and dusky scent to oils, though most people use the intensely scented flowers.

Common, or English, lavender is renowned for its soothing effects. Its scent calms the nervous system, and its oil reduces scar tissue formation from burns; many herbalists include the essential oil of lavender in healing salves.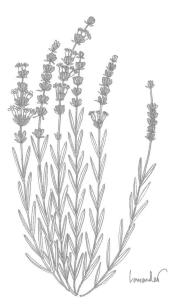

But don't let its beauty and sweet scent fool you: the distilled oil is antibacterial and antiseptic and has been listed in the United States Pharmacopoeia–National Formulary since 1820. Lavender essential oil kills diphtheria bacilli, typhoid bacilli, streptococci, and pneumococci.

 You'll find lavender recipes and formulas in the following chapters:

Chapter 6. For Infant and Child
Children's Sleepytime Tonic

LEMON BALM
Melissa officinalis

This amazing garden or container plant has been a perennial favorite of herbalists and gardeners for centuries. Growing in large mounds or tall "cushions" of upright stalks, this mint family member boasts the typical rough, oval leaves and tiny, unassuming white flowers associated with mints in general. I've grown thick mounds of lemon balm whose leaves are dark green and thick like leather, as well as tall, airy lemon balm whose leaves are thin and wispy. Either way, when the leaves are rubbed or crushed, they release the classic lemony scent that brought this humble herb world-class fame.

Lemon balm is renowned for its effect on the nervous system and is often included by knowledgeable herbalists in remedies for attention deficit disorder, attention-deficit/hyperactivity disorder, manic depressive disorder, depression, and obsessive compulsive disorder. Simply smelling the citrusy herb in the summer is enough to provide a calm feeling of contentment and a certain clarity, and it has become the favorite of test takers who rely on its volatile oils to stir memory and awaken the brain. I like to think of lemon balm as the patron flower of teachers and mentors, hovering over their heads to impart knowledge, wisdom, and kindness. She makes words clear, streamlines thoughts, and helps ideas explode.

Lemon balm also has an affinity for the digestive system and works well for gas, dyspepsia, or ulcers due to nervousness.

This herb infuses well in oil—which I include in my Lemon Balm Salve (*balm* is the true word here)—and can be used for burns, dry skin, and cold sores. It is antiviral and should be included in every cold and flu remedy. The leaves contain essential oils and other highly volatile principles; when harvesting, you need to dry it carefully in the shade on flat screens, but be sure to use only fresh leaves for tinctures.

You'll find lemon balm recipes and formulas in the following chapters:

Chapter 5. For the Expectant and New Mother
Holly's Organic Mother's Tea
New Mother's Transition Formula
Happy Sun Tea

Chapter 6. For Infant and Child
Children's Digestive Glycerite
Lemon Balm Infusion

Lemon Balm

THE MINTS: PEPPERMINT AND SPEARMINT
Mentha piperita and *Mentha spicata*

I first met wild mint during a countryside excursion on, of all things, a real-estate jaunt. Some friends and I were harboring fantasies of buying mountain property, and we visited a beautiful south-facing valley for sale near Boone, North Carolina. The gorgeous land consisted of several hundred acres bordered by tall hemlock- and maple-covered ridges, and the valley in between harbored remnants of the previous century's farm and the wilderness before that. We found old sheds, the original garden grown over with goldenrod, and rare wildflowers on the top ridge. Along a creek, we came upon colonies of wild spearmint that had likely escaped from cultivation decades earlier; we munched on this and inhaled its sweet aroma as we returned to the car and real life. Here on Martha's Vineyard, I've discovered another wild mint altogether—a blue-gray variety bearing little resemblance to the lush, green wild spearmint but sharing that pungent scent. I believe this mint might be grey mint (*Mentha vagans*), though I can find no reference to it in any of my field guides. Surely it's been a favorite of the native Wampanoag tribe for generations, for its smell is intensely aromatic, and it forms lovely, gray seed balls at the top in November.

When I use mint, I often feel a certain energy, like an electrical charge, a current that runs in every direction, a zippy connection to some higher source. Many people feel a refreshing rush of energy from the scent and flavor of mint, which has made this common "weed" one of the world's most frequently used; it appears in diverse culinary and medicinal applications from Morocco (it's a staple in the delicious green tea) to Mexico (*herba buena* is that country's mint of choice for healing salves). Because of the zingy quality we feel when we consume mint, I like to say it is the Buddha of the plant world, the bodhisattva, the healer who can transport us toward knowledge and wisdom. And, of course, it makes a great tea.

The most common types are native wild, or field, mint (*Mentha arvensis*) and escaped-from-cultivation peppermint and spearmint. All mints are easy to recognize simply by their shape and smell: they grow in thick mats, using long, thin runner roots to spread and establish new plants; they all have square stems (not round); their leaves are generally small ovals with tiny serrations on the edges; and they obviously smell minty in some way. There are many varieties of mint, which come in dozens of scents from wintergreen to lemon to chocolate to apple, but in this book, I use only spearmint and peppermint. Peppermint is generally sharper, while spearmint is sweeter. In general, they can be used interchangeably, though I find spearmint more useful as a tea for children's complaints and digestive upset and as a tea blend ingredient; I use peppermint in tinctures for digestive upset and circulatory remedies. Both are good for relieving anxiety and maintaining focus. Catnip (catmint) and motherwort are also mints, but because they have unique medicinal uses, they are referred to specifically by name throughout this book.

I always recommend mint when people ask for a good erosion-control plant. Peppermint is ideal, because it grows in poor, sandy, and well-drained soils; spreads rapidly; and puts out a great root system that holds loose soil in place, even on hillsides and banks. It also attracts bees and other pollinators; produces lovely, violet-colored flowers; and holds its green leaves for an extended period during the growing season. It is both edible and medicinal.

Medicinally, mint is a wonderful colic remedy for babies, a soothing stomach-ache reliever for children, and a cure for flatulent dyspepsia. It relieves nausea and the desire to vomit. Mint is one of those rare plants that is both warming and cooling; as a warming and rejuvenating herb, it encourages circulatory flow, which is useful to treat chronic lethargy, cardiac illness, and mild depression. As a cooling herb, it soothes sunburned skin and brews into a wonderful iced tea for cooling off on hot summer days. It is a great addition to internal remedies for the common cold, fever, and influenza, as well as external remedies for wounds, topical ulcers, and scrapes. Since it rejuvenates as it soothes, mint makes a fabulous foot balm. It also makes a lovely syrup—easy, tasty, and useful as a tea sweetener and medicine-cabinet staple.

I find myself making iced peppermint tea in the summer (see the recipe for Menemsha Mint Tea in chapter 13: Tummy Health), and who can resist hot peppermint tea in the winter? Add a peppermint candy stick to hot chocolate or a spoonful of peppermint syrup to any kind of tea.

Mint is antibacterial, antiseptic, carminative, mildly anesthetic, analgesic, and nervine, which is a tonic to the nervous system. And of course, it is a delicious food, high in vitamin A with a moderate vitamin C content.

You'll find peppermint/spearmint recipes and formulas in the following chapters:

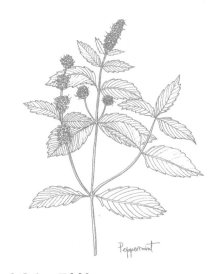

Peppermint

NETTLE
Urtica dioica

Long hailed as a fiber plant for making durable linen in Scotland and many third-world countries, nettle (sometimes known as "stinging nettle") has also befriended humanity with its storehouse of vitamins and minerals. It makes one of the most nutritive tonics available. In need of calcium, magnesium, trace minerals, protein, and chlorophyll? Look no further. This herb has them. Mineral-rich nettle treats anemia and is valuable during pregnancy, breast-feeding, and menopause. And we are now learning that the root serves a primary function in the treatment of prostate inflammation.

Nettle can also be used as a hair rinse. The "doctrine of signature" convinced people in the Middle Ages that because nettle is covered with fine hairs, it could serve as a hair tonic. Indeed, nettle makes a wonderful strengthening rinse for dark hair.

The hairs on the plant contain irritating formic acid, and because of its sting, it has been used externally to treat arthritis. The acid burns and causes blood to flow to the area to speed healing; the area becomes inflamed, which is why nettle is called a rubefacient. This old-fashioned process is termed *urtication* from nettle's genus name, *Urtica*.

You can enjoy the many benefits of this herb without getting stung. Simply wear gloves to collect fresh nettle and either dry it or steam it; both methods deactivate the formic acid. When I lived in the rugged wilds of eastern Tennessee, our log cabin sat on a knoll in a deep valley above the Wautaga River. My husband, Rocco, and I would occasionally hike down to the wet bottomlands by the river's edge to harvest one- to two-foot-high nettles. Our boots sank in the muck, hawks flew over the rapids beside us, and we were sometimes stung by the nettles' hairs, but it was worth it. Once we dried our treasure, we could brew earthy nettle tea all year long. I like to think of nettle as a gnome of sorts, living happily low to the wet earth. Look for nettle on rich, wet, mucky riverbanks while enjoying the scent of earth right after a rain.

If you're cultivating nettle, grow it in rich soil in the shade. It is best harvested when it is less than a foot high; once it grows to human height, it's too tough and fibrous to make a good food, though it can still be brewed for tea. (I love steamed nettles with vinegar, and beloved herbalist Euell Gibbons recommended nettle puree and nettle pudding.) Nettle leaves are somewhat oval—broad in the middle and narrowing to a sharp tip. The stalks are tall, strong, and succulent, and both the leaves and the stalk are covered with fine, sharp, stinging hairs. The flowers are easiest to identify, as they look like miniature explosions of off-white, little crazy rays from a tiny white firecracker. These flowers explode from every axil where the leaf meets the stalk. In most field guides, the flowers are listed as "green."

To harvest the fresh plant, use gloves to snip off the leaves or cut the stalk at the base; you can use the entire aboveground plant. Steam or dry it immediately. When purchasing dried nettle, make sure the herb is a rich, dark green (not light green) and that it smells earthy.

 You'll find nettle recipes and formulas in the following chapters:

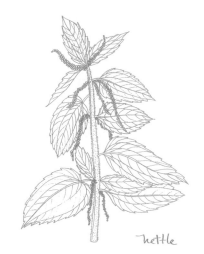
nettle

PLANTAIN
Plantago major, P. lanceolata

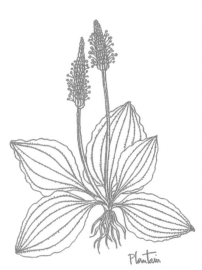

Plantain

One of my all-time favorite herbs for making medicines is plantain, a common weed throughout much of the western hemisphere. It is so common, in fact, that it enjoys many names, including Englishman's foot—everywhere colonists trod in the New World, plantain would sprout. This herb is easily recognizable with its two types of leaves: large-leaf plantain boasts wide, oval-shaped leaves that grow from a single "rosette," while lance-leaf plantain has long, narrow leaves. In each case, long, parallel ridges, or veins, run down the length of the leaf. In poor, compacted soil, the plants stay low to the ground and have small leaves the size of a quarter, but in rich soil, they can grow upward of two feet with leaves broader than your outstretched hand. In the fall, they put out seed stalks that grow tall and skinny with a one-inch tip of tiny seeds on the end.

My early mentor, Georgia Gillis in the North Carolina mountains, called it "PLAN-uhn," and she showed me how to pluck a leaf; chew it; and apply it to a thorn, splinter, or bee sting. In turn, many years later, I introduced it to my friend Sarah from Ireland, who was searching for a remedy for her mother's bug bites. She showed it to her mother, who exclaimed, "Icky yacky? That's what we call this plant in County Wexford! I had no idea it was good for anything."

Well, I can see why this plant might be called icky yacky, because it is rather viscous when steeped in water, feels gummy in the mouth, and is rather tasteless. When dry, it's stringy and fibrous. But that's the whole beauty of it: those large oval or spear-shaped leaves are full of mucilage and strings, and these are the parts that are useful. Herbalists prize plantain for its beneficial effects on the digestive tract, since it soothes stomach upset, peptic ulcer, gastritis, and heartburn. We also call on it for its stringiness, because when it's chewed, macerated, or chopped and then placed on the skin, it has the miraculous ability to draw poisons and objects such as splinters from the skin and heal tissue.

This fantastic drawing agent was used in old-fashioned "drawing salves." Immediately after my husband got a tattoo on his shoulder, his skin was sore, so being the wonderful wife that I am, I applied a handmade salve to the spot. Much to our surprise, fresh tattoo ink began rising to the surface! The plantain was drawing it out. Needless to say, I quickly wiped it off. Bee and snake venom, bug bites, splinters, and (according to some) even cysts and tumors can be coaxed from beneath the upper layer of flesh and removed with the constant application of plantain (and other drawing herbs such as poke root).

Plantain leaf's gentle astringency makes it useful for treating hemorrhoids (externally) and, when taken internally as a tea, for treating bronchitis and diarrhea.

Plantain is also a wild edible, specifically as a wilderness emergency food. Although palatable, it requires some getting used to. When young, the tiny leaves make a decent addition to spring salads with wood sorrel, lamb's quarter, watercress, early lettuce, branch lettuce, and jewelweed sprouts. Even better than the leaves are the seeds. In autumn, the mature seeds grow at the top of the seed stalk and are commonly employed as missiles by children in serious attempts at warfare. These edible seeds may be collected and sprinkled over your morning oatmeal in much the same way as textured vegetable protein (TVP) or wheat bran. They are highly nutritious and contain a fair amount of mucilage, so they soothe the stomach lining as well. You can eat the seeds raw or gently roast and store them for winter.

 You'll find plantain recipes and formulas in the following chapters:

Chapter 5. For the Expectant and New Mother
Herby Sitz Bath

Chapter 6. For Infant and Child
Cradle Cap Oil
Baby Scalp Rinse
Children's Raspberry Formula with Yarrow
Children's Digestive Glycerite

Chapter 7. Especially for Women
Cyst-Dissolving Oil

Chapter 8. Especially for Men
Prostate Suppository

Chapter 10. Sniffles, Colds, and Viruses
Wild Weed Cough Brew

Chapter 11. Healing Wounds
Rosemary's Blessing First Aid Ointment
Quick Plantain Poultice
Red Clover Bee Sting Cream

Marshmallow-Plantain Burn Remedy
Magical Jewelweed-Plantain Cubes
Jewelweed Poison Ivy Spray

RASPBERRY
Rubus idaeus, R. strigosus

Red raspberries, of course, are the delicious little cap-shaped berries that we all love to pick from the briar bush and pop in our mouths. Less well known are those green-on-top-silver-underneath, lightly fuzzy leaves that have been used for centuries by Wise Women as a uterine strengthener.

As many herbalists say, these leaves have an "affinity" for the uterus. They contain high (for plants) levels of calcium, which is wonderful for building bone mass in a pregnant or lactating woman. They also contain enough tannin and tart (citric and malic) acids to be slightly astringent, and this astringency promotes a nice, tight uterus that's ready to hold on to and shelter a growing baby. Raspberry leaves tighten things up and keep them shipshape.

I like to think of raspberry as a Mary Poppins midwife: she sweeps, mops, and scours but always with a soft flannel cloth. Herbalists use raspberry to keep the uterus and cervix strong, as its regular use during the third trimester of pregnancy can tone the womb for a successful delivery and keep the risk of hemorrhage low. You can drink a strong raspberry infusion during labor, suck on raspberry ice cubes (made from the infusion), or take a raspberry leaf tincture.

Raspberry can also be used externally, making a wonderful addition to a postpartum sitz bath. It tightens tissues, reduces muscle spasms, and relieves soreness. It also contributes to healthy milk production and eases leucorrhoea (a heavy, white vaginal discharge some women experience due to increased estrogen).

Raspberry plants can, of course, be distinguished from blackberry by the berries; but also by the size and color of the canes. Blackberry canes are thin and solid green, while raspberry canes are thicker and a silvery blue color. Blackberry leaves are solid green on both the top and the bottom, while raspberry leaves are pale, fuzzy green on top but silver underneath. When harvesting, pick only first-year leaves and lay them flat on a screen or newspaper to dry. The leaves can be harvested throughout the season.

 You'll find recipes and formulas using raspberry in the following chapters:

Chapter 5. For the Expectant and New Mother
Sweet Raspberry Calcium Brew
Red Raspberry Pregnancy Tonic Infusion
Raspberry Sparkle Beverage
Mother's Meadow Tea
Holly's Organic Mother's Tea
Wild Yam Infusion
Morning Sickness Tincture
Breast Milk Fountain Tea

Chapter 6. For Infant and Child
Children's Raspberry Formula with Yarrow

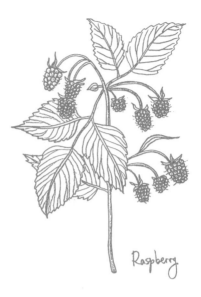

Raspberry

RED CLOVER
Trifolium pratense

Who doesn't adore red clover? Children love this wildflower instinctively because it is sweet tasting and beautiful. Perhaps clover seems like the sweet aunt who shows up in a pink shirt, light purple sweater, and funky green earrings, doling out treasures from her travels. She's fresh and sweet and easy. Gardeners treasure clover and its cousins as valuable nitrogen fixers for the soil, and you'll find it scattered among the grasses and weeds of rich meadows.

Red clover carries a reddish-pink globe flower directly on top of three little leaves; this set of blossom and leaf is called the "clover top." In its Latin name,

Trifolium refers to the three leaves, and *pratense* means it lives in the meadow. It grows on long, skinny stems and often blooms again in late summer after its first appearance in early summer—meaning you can harvest it twice.

Long esteemed as a tasty tea flower, red clover is a powerhouse of a medicine. The blossoms are gathered to make both internal and external remedies to treat cases of eczema and psoriasis in children and adults. In folk medicine, red clover is widely regarded for treating skin cancers, and recent evidence shows that it contains antineoplastic beta-sitosterol, which inhibits cancerous growths. One of my favorite herbalists, the nineteenth-century renegade healer Samuel Thompson, used red clover in a paste to treat skin cancers, and today it is often found in treatments for breast cancer.

Red clover is frequently used to address the female hormonal system and is included in fertility formulas and menopausal remedies for hot flashes and vaginal dryness. I like to include it in preparations for teenage girls, as it is balancing and sweet. Taken as a whole-plant infusion, this medicine is much safer than synthetic estrogen drugs and more holistically balanced. I recommend a red clover infusion douche for cervical dysplasia and red clover teas or tinctures for chronic conditions such as pelvic inflammatory disease, amenorrhea, and infertility.

Red clover is mild enough for children to drink as a tea to address eczema from the inside out. (Also experiment with diet to determine if eczema rashes are caused by an allergen, often dairy or wheat.) It also makes a fabulous skin remedy when used in a poultice, compress, oil, or salve. For example, a compress with tea made from red clover blossoms is useful for burns, weepy rashes, and blisters; an oil infused from the blossoms can be used to treat sore nipples and dry lips. Combined with specific eczema and psoriasis herbs such as pau d'arco and calendula, red clover lends a gentle but effective hand to cleaning and healing the skin.

It's renowned as a blood cleanser, lymph drainer, and circulatory aid, and it is frequently included in herbal blends for toxin removal. I find it combines well with calendula, violet, and rose in topical preparations and with black cohosh, elder flower, and blue vervain in internal formulas.

You'll find recipes and formulas containing red clover in the following chapters:

Chapter 5. For the Expectant and New Mother
Herby Sitz Bath
Breast Milk Fountain Tea
Nipple Nurse Salve 2

Chapter 6. For Infant and Child
Cradle Cap Oil
Baby Scalp Rinse
Calendula-Beeswax Salve
Baby Massage Oil

Chapter 7. Especially for Women
Delicious Mineral Infusion
Nipple Moisturizing Oil
Cyst Dissolving Oil
Love Your Lymph System Tea
Wild Herbflower Tea
Fertili-Tea
Lovely Hormone Tea
Menopause Friend Tincture

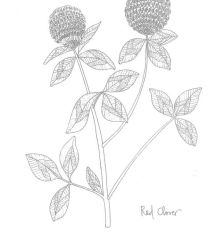

Red Clover

Chapter 9. Everyday Tonics for Vitality
Everyday Immune Tonic
Women's Everyday Tonic Tea

Chapter 10. For Sniffles, Colds, and Viruses
Elderberry-Ginger Syrup for Colds and Flu
Antiviral Tincture

Chapter 11. Healing Wounds
Rosemary's Blessing First Aid Ointment

ROSE
Rosa spp.

Countless generations have celebrated the rose. Cleopatra was said to have scented the sails of her barge with rose petals and strewn them about the floors of her palace; the Greek herbalist Dioscorides used rose petal paste and powder for specific ailments; Homer gave Aphrodite oil of rose petal to cure Hector's wounds in *The Iliad;* and Shakespeare wrote sonnet after sonnet and play after play with references to his beloved flower. From Pliny to Nero to Empress Josephine, humanity has long been in love with roses for their beauty and captivating scent. There are hundreds of cultivated varieties and a number of lovely wild varieties in the United States, most of which descend from only four varieties cultivated centuries ago. Historically, roses were abundant in Egypt, Anatolia (Turkey), China, and eventually all over the Roman Empire and Europe, holding a solid place in apothecaries and hospitals.

But beauty and scent aside, there is a lot of medicine to be found in a rose bush. The hips (those red sacs that appear after the flower falls) are packed with vitamin C that can easily be consumed in a tea, syrup, or jam; nearly two thousand years ago, Dioscorides recommended rose hips as a cure for coughing up blood. For centuries, the petals and unopened buds have been used for syrups and eyewashes, and I also use the petals frequently in my herbal formulas for women and teenagers to allay anxiety. The seventeenth-century herbalist Nicholas Culpeper celebrated the syrups and conserves made from both the petals and the hips, remedies still made today to address a variety of physical and emotional problems. Rose is a transcendent herb that can remind us of our changing human nature: we blossom, yet our luster fades. We can send out thorns, yet like rose petals, we can rub soft as blush against a baby's cheek.

Recipes throughout this book show how to take the fragrant flower blossoms and turn them into healing tinctures, teas, and syrups. Harvest only those blossoms you are certain have not been sprayed with pesticides or herbicides.

 You'll find rose recipes and formulas in the following chapters:

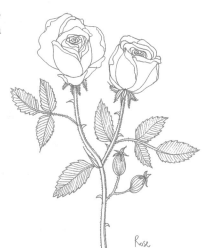

Chapter 5. For the Expectant and New Mother
New Mother's Transition Tea
Elder Flower Hydrosol Spritzer
Nipple Nurse Salve 2

Chapter 6. For Infant and Child
Katama Chamomile Calming Blend Tea

Rose

YARROW
Achillea millefolium

One of my favorite plants, yarrow is a versatile and necessary friend for herbal healing. It's used in myriad ways: staunching bleeding wounds, healing cuts and scrapes, and treating colds and flu. Sometimes called field pepper (for its rejuvenating scent), yarrow grows to about hip height; boasts feathery leaves up and down the stalk; and blooms heartily with one to three creamy white, flat-topped umbels of tiny flowers. The stalk is stiff and straight and, I've been told, has been used in Asia for divination purposes per the I Ching.

Yarrow works in different ways, depending on the way you prepare it. For instance, brewing a hot tea of yarrow leaves or flowers will induce sweating (it's a diaphoretic); this will often break fevers. In this capacity, yarrow combines well with elder flower and ginger. Brewing it in a tea and drinking it cold will stimulate the need to urinate (it's a diuretic). This is useful if you suffer from a urinary tract or kidney infection, because the herb flushes out the system, at the same time bringing its germ-fighting and astringent properties to the area. This is also useful for treating colds and influenza, since the urinary system flush rids the body of excess and damaging material.

But that's not all. Yarrow is wonderfully useful in topical preparations to fight skin infections, heal wounds, and stop bleeding. Because yarrow is astringent, it is beneficial to take it (as tea or tincture) during diarrhea since it helps retain water. Similarly, it contracts tissues in the gut, which leads to the expulsion of gas during gastritis. For minor stomach ulcers, its astringency can help stop bleeding. Legend has it that the Greek hero Achilles favored yarrow and used it to heal the wounds of his soldiers.

Add yarrow leaves to your bitters recipes and include it in cough syrups and (sparingly) in wintertime teas.

 You'll find yarrow recipes and formulas in the following chapters:

Chapter 5. For the Expectant and New Mother
Herby Sitz Bath
"No More Dairy Queen" Breast Milk Drying Formula

Chapter 6. For Infant and Child
Children's Raspberry Formula with Yarrow

Chapter 7. Especially for Women
Calendula Suppository

Chapter 8. Especially for Men
"Get to the Root of the Problem" Prostate Tonic
Men's Grounding Formula
Foot Soak

Chapter 10. Sniffles, Colds, and Viruses
West Chop Winter Tea for Colds and Flu
Elderberry-Ginger Syrup for Colds and Flu

Chapter 11. Healing Wounds
Rosemary's Blessing First Aid Ointment
Quick Yarrow Compress
Jewelweed Poison Ivy Spray

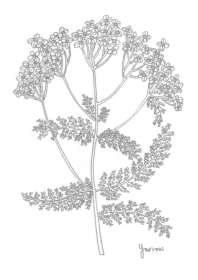

Yarrow

Through patient experimentation, observation, and a sense of adventure, you'll find yourself truly enjoying these thirteen Essential Herbs and returning to them time and again to help with physical and emotional needs. My hope is that these herbs will start to feel like old friends: present and available, helpful and useful, beautiful in their wisdom and familiarity.

Now that you can identify them and have a sense of their history, what can you do with them? Our herbal heritage abounds with beloved recipes for making foods, medicines, and other delights with these plants. The following chapters will guide you through the basics of making herbal medicines and also the specifics for using these particular herbs.

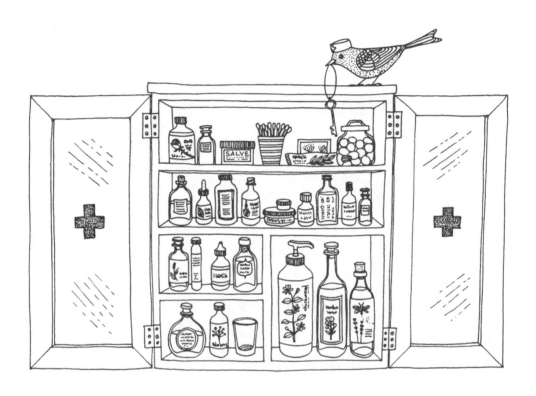

Part Two

—————∘⫯∘—————

THE ART OF HERBAL
MEDICINE MAKING

Where the spirit does not work with the hand, there is no art.

—Leonardo da Vinci

Chapter Three

INTRODUCING HERBAL
MEDICINE MAKING

I found entering herbalism as a handcrafter to be a return to roots, if you'll pardon the expression—a return to the recognition of the beauty, simplicity, and utility of nature's bounty. I think nature likes that we make things from her. She's given us the colors, the textures, and the flavors; all we have to do is assemble them to meet our notion of "right" and use them. We do this readily with food, chopping and blending and mixing until the final dish resembles our idea of perfection. It's just a short hop to do the same with medicine.

Medicine making need not be complicated or time-consuming. The act of combining ingredients to create delicious teas, potent tinctures, creamy salves, energizing elixirs, and tasty syrups is a rewarding experience—and an important part of the healing process. As wildcrafter Euell Gibbons, someone I consider a beloved influence, said, "Food should never be merely nourishment, a means of keeping us alive, but should be one of the amenities that make life a joy." Similarly, herbal remedies should be not only medicine, a means of rescue from disease, but also and foremost a means of sustenance, joy, and connection with the living world around us.

Medicine comes in a variety of forms and from a variety of sources. The first, naturally, is nature. Ridding ourselves of the fallacy that real medicine is found only in bottles packaged with expiration dates or wrapped in colorful cardboard boxes on a retail store shelf is the first step toward understanding the real value of healing. True healing is an organic experience that involves not only our senses of taste, touch, and smell but also our sense of purpose and of being fulfilled. Self-fulfillment includes being self-sufficient, creative, and free to explore and learn—values easily incorporated into making herbal medicines for a healthy lifestyle. Harvesting and/or making remedies gives us a sense of self-sufficiency, and the creativity that comes from experimenting (with herbs as both food and medicine) is a healing force in itself. The freedom to explore nature and learn about our collective herbal heritage can contribute to a sense of purpose, regardless of our career or professional path.

Medicine making can be straightforward or wonderfully intricate; indeed, the formulas in this book range from fun and simple to involved but highly rewarding. I suggest clearing off a shelf or section of your kitchen that will be dedicated to your creations. Store them at eye level in a single row, so their colors (and labels) are visible. This way they won't get lost in the shuffle of closets and boxes, and you'll be able to reach out and use them daily for health, vitality, and nourishment. That's the fun thing about crafting herbal medicines: your own energy has gone into the creation of functional treasures meant for the healing and well-being of you and your family.

I recommend that people make their own remedies for a variety of reasons:

- The remedies are surprisingly simple and can be made before they're needed. For instance, travelers can make Digestive Aid/Gas Relief

Tincture before traveling, and mothers-to-be can prepare a blend of dried Mother's Meadow Tea herbs during pregnancy.

- It's a rewarding experience to learn about plants instead of relying on store-bought preparations. Connecting with plants is a huge part of healing and is a peaceful and heartening experience.
- Children who witness you harvesting plants will want to do the same. They will also establish relationships with the plants and consider this process as completely natural. They'll think, "Of course we connect with plants. Of course we love the earth. It's what we do, because Mommy and Daddy do it." My son Gabriel accompanies me on herb walks, forever running ahead and calling back, "Mom! Here's a sassafras," or "Watch your step, I just found a patch of Indian pipe!" Mother Nature influenced this child early, and I believe his life will be long and rich with the magic of the natural world.
- What you can make at home is far superior to what you can purchase in a typical store. Dried herbs sold in stores (especially in capsules) have often been sitting in a warehouse until the remedy is no longer potent. Dried herbs have a shelf life of one year; if it's too old, it simply won't work. Harvesting and preparing your own plants assures you that each plant is indeed the one you believe it to be, that it is grown without pesticides, and that it is potent.

Don't be discouraged if the first dose of your fresh, wonderful, new medicine doesn't give discernable results. The best results come from consistent and dedicated use; herbal medicine is not a "magic bullet," and it can sometimes take many doses before you notice changes. Have faith; consistent use will show you what your medicine is made of and will give your body time to adjust and respond appropriately.

Chapter Four

MEDICINE-MAKING METHODS

With familiarity, curiosity, and patience, we can make strangers into friends and wild weeds into healing remedies. A number of competent herbalists and healers have shared the following guidelines with me, and these guidelines consistently make effective remedies that can be used over and over again. Refer to them often when making remedies; see pages 287–90 for dosage information.

NECESSARY EQUIPMENT

Over the course of sixteen years, I've accumulated a supply of equipment, tools, and props that help me make herbal concoctions safely, efficiently, and with minimal destruction of other kitchen gadgets. Because herbal medicine making is fun, basic, and essentially a kitchen activity, the equipment you need is often already at hand or easy to acquire.

Be sure you have the following equipment that can be shared equally between general kitchen duty and medicine making:

Stockpot
Saucepan
Canning jars

Large bowls
Long-handled spoons and regular spoons
Spatulas
Chopping block and sharp knives
Thin sticks or skewers
Sieves and strainers
Teapot

You also need to stock your crafts pantry with dedicated equipment to be used only for herbal medicine making. Beeswax is nearly impossible to remove from most surfaces, and certain herbs stain wood, plastic, and even porcelain, so the following items must be purchased exclusively for medicine making (you can often find them inexpensively at yard sales and thrift stores).

Spice/coffee grinder
Cutting board for beeswax
Knife for cutting beeswax
Glass measuring cup for salve making
Metal measuring cup for salve making
Canning jar lids
Rubber spatula
Sieves and strainers
A deep kettle or soup pot
Aluminum foil

THE HOME APOTHECARY: CRAFTING INSTRUCTIONS

There are as many ways to make herbal medicines as there are herbalists. I've attended workshops with those who measure and weigh to the nth degree, those who purchase materials and liquids only from certified organic family farms, those who steep on the full moon and decant on the new moon, those who steep on the full moon and decant on the next full moon, those who steep on the full moon and don't decant for a whole year, and finally those who throw together whatever they have at hand and eyeball the measurement to their liking. This last method is the closest to the folk method of healing, and it is closest to my heart.

My formulas are generally somewhere in the middle—they are simple to make and measure, yet they are made with the highest-quality ingredients and in concert with lunar energies. Part of the joy of herbalism is experimenting and discovering what works, what doesn't, and how the plants respond to processing. Making medicines is partly scientific, partly intuitive. Don't be afraid to combine methods to suit your needs and discover what works for you. For a complete and comprehensive guide to professional medicine making, see James Green's *The Herbal Medicine-Maker's Handbook*. For simpler folk methods and recipes for family healing, see Rosemary Gladstar's *Family Herbal* or Susun Weed's *Healing Wise*. The methods they describe, along with my own, provide high-quality herbal medicines using intuition, science, nature, and mathematics—all to a greater or lesser degree.

Tinctures and Tincture-Based Medicines

A *tincture* is a concentrated liquid extract of a healing plant that is meant to be taken as an internal medicine. It can be made from any part of the plant (leaves, seeds, roots, bark, flowers, stem), and although it takes some time to make, the finished tincture is a quick and convenient medicine, often preferred by busy mothers for its ease of use.

Generally, tinctures require one or more liquids as the menstruum (carrier). These liquids generally include grain alcohol such as vodka, brandy, or wine (but not rubbing or isopropyl alcohol, which are for external use only!); vegetable glycerin (a sweet-tasting by-product of the soap-making industry that has a viscous consistency); apple cider vinegar; or distilled (some herbalists call it "thirsty") water. Other menstruums are oil and distilled witch hazel, which are covered in later sections in this chapter.

Making an Alcohol Tincture

The standard herbal method for making an alcohol-based tincture is to use fresh plant material with a ratio of one part herb to two parts liquid (1:2); dried plants require a less concentrated ratio (1:5). This makes a potent, usable, and balanced medicine. If you're new to making tinctures, practice using one part of one herb at a time; for example, tincture only plantain leaves or only calendula flowers. Combine more herbs later as your expertise grows.

To make the tincture, gather dried herbs or harvest fresh ones, strip the usable parts from the stems or branches, and chop them thoroughly to get the most surface area. (Some herbalists recommend blending the herbs and the menstruum together in a blender or Vitamix, but I find this introduces too much air into the product and can lead to spoilage. Coarsely chopping the herbs with a knife is sufficient.)

REMOVING ALCOHOL CONTENT

There are two ways to remove the alcohol content of a tincture. One is to gently heat the tincture, one cup at a time, in a saucepan. The heat causes the alcohol to evaporate, so you need to add sufficient glycerin to replace the alcohol. The potency of the tincture will be slightly reduced.

I prefer the following method: when you use the tincture, drop the appropriate dosage (in number of drops or teaspoons) into a cup of hot water or tea. Let it sit for two minutes so the alcohol can evaporate (most of it will). Drink the tea.

Place the herb(s) in a clean, dry, 1-quart glass jar. Pack the jar tight and nearly full if you are using fresh herbs; if you're using dried, pack the jar one-third full.

Prepare the menstruum (liquid). For a fresh herb–alcohol tincture, the menstruum is usually 100 percent grain alcohol (190 proof). For a dried herb–alcohol tincture, more water is acceptable and 40 proof or 50 proof alcohol is fine. The choice of menstruum also depends on the herb: hard substances such as echinacea root and milk thistle seeds require a stronger alcohol concentration, whereas softer plant materials such as violet flower require a milder concentration.

INTUITIVE MEDICINE MAKING

Though scientists claim that 190 proof alcohol is essential to fresh herb tinctures, I disagree. Intuition sometimes tells us what scientists might balk at but will later come to recognize as valid. I often tincture more delicate fresh herbs—such as violet flower, lemon balm, or rose petal—in brandy or a low-proof vodka. Use whatever method feels appropriate to you, and don't be intimidated into using a stronger alcohol than you feel is justified. Just be sure the product is well preserved and will resist bacterial growth.

Pour the menstruum into the jar using a long, thin stick, a wooden-handled spoon, or a skewer to poke around the sides to release air bubbles. Fill to within ¼ inch of the rim of the jar. Clean the rim, and cap the jar tightly.

Label it in two locations. On two pieces of masking tape write the name of the herb(s), the date, and the menstruum used. Place one piece of tape on the lid and one on the side of the jar. Place the jar in a cool, dark cabinet. Shake it daily for two to four weeks.

Decant (strain) the liquid into a clean container and press the herbs firmly to release as much valuable liquid as possible. Compost the leftover herbs. Bottle the tincture; label it; and store it in a cool, dark cabinet.

It will have a shelf life of approximately eight to ten years.

Making a Glycerin Tincture

Glycerin tinctures are suitable for more delicate plant parts, such as flower petals and blossoms, and for people with a sensitivity to alcohol. This technique differs from that for an alcohol tincture in that only vegetable glycerin and water are used as the menstruum. I generally avoid making 100 percent glycerin tinctures because they have a shorter shelf life (since they aren't preserved with alcohol) and because glycerin doesn't pull all the desired chemicals from the plant. I often use a one-third method with one-third vodka, one-third glycerin, and one-third water instead of a straight glycerin-water mixture.

To make the tincture, gather dried herbs or harvest fresh ones, strip the usable parts from the stems or branches, and chop them thoroughly to get the most surface area. (Some herbalists recommend blending the herbs and the menstruum together in a blender or Vitamix, but I find this introduces too much air into the product and can lead to spoilage.)

Place the herb(s) in a clean, dry, 1-quart glass jar. Pack the jar tight and nearly full if you are using fresh herbs; if you're using dried, pack the jar one-third full.

Prepare the menstruum (liquid) by combining ½ quart vegetable glycerin with ½ quart distilled water. Whisk this combination together in a separate container.

Pour the menstruum into the jar, using a long, thin stick, a wooden-handled spoon, or a skewer to poke around the sides to release air bubbles. Fill to within ¼ inch of the rim of the jar. Clean the rim, and cap the jar tightly.

Label it in two locations. On two pieces of masking tape write the name of the herb(s), the date, and the menstruum used. Place one piece of tape on the lid and one on the side of the jar. Place the jar in a cool, dark cabinet. Shake it daily for two to four weeks.

Decant (strain) the liquid into a clean container and press the herbs firmly to release as much valuable liquid as possible. Compost the leftover herbs. Bottle the tincture; label it; and store it in a cool, dark cabinet.

It will have a shelf life of approximately two years.

YES, LABEL THAT JAR!

Labeling is important, even though it takes extra time. From experience, I know the heartache of finding a beautiful jar of tincture in the back of the cabinet and having no idea what's in it. Put a strip of masking tape on both the lid and the side of the jar and write the name of the plant, the menstruum, and the date you made it. Don't place a sticky note on the lid; it will invariably fall off.

Making a Vinegar Tincture

A vinegar tincture differs from alcohol or glycerin tinctures in several ways. Vinegar is used primarily with herbs or roots that are high in iron and other minerals, as the vinegar easily pulls these minerals from the herbal material. Because it is made from apples, apple cider vinegar is a safe food and can be consumed by children or elderly people with ease and confidence. Vinegar is naturally rich in enzymes and nutritious. A vinegar tincture has a shorter shelf life and will typically last only six months to a year—not the eight to ten years of an alcohol tincture. When preparing a vinegar menstruum, you must always gently heat the vinegar in a saucepan first. This heating action draws a greater concentration of minerals from the plant material, resulting in a stronger medicine.

To make the tincture, gather dried or harvest fresh herbs or roots, such as dandelion leaves or roots, yellow dock root, or burdock roots. Wash the herbs well. Chop them thoroughly to get the most surface area. (Some herbalists recommend blending the herbs and the menstruum together in a blender or Vitamix, but I find this introduces too much air into the product and can lead to spoilage.)

Place the herbs in a clean, dry, 1-quart glass jar. Pack the jar tight and nearly full if you are using fresh herbs; if you're using dried, pack the jar one-fifth to one-third full.

Prepare the menstruum (liquid). In a small saucepan, gently heat 2 cups vinegar to simmering, but don't let it boil. Add 2 cups distilled water and stir gently.

Pour the menstruum into the jar, using a long, thin stick, a wooden-handled spoon, or a skewer to poke around the sides to release air bubbles. Fill to within $1/4$ inch of the rim of the jar. Clean the rim and cap the jar tightly with a plastic lid (a metal lid will react with the vinegar and rust).

Label it in two locations. On two pieces of masking tape write the name of the herb(s), the date, and the menstruum used. Place one piece of tape on the lid and one on the side of the jar. Place the jar in a cool, dark cabinet on top of a plate. This is important, because the vinegar solution can ooze up out of the cap and ruin counters, cabinets, and shelves. Shake the jar daily for two to four weeks.

Decant (strain) the liquid and press the herbs firmly to get out as much valuable liquid as possible. Compost the leftover herbs. Bottle the tincture; label it; and store it in a cool, dark cabinet.

It will have a shelf life of approximately six to twelve months.

Oils and Oil-Based Medicines

Though oils are made in a similar process, their creation is a bit different from that of other tinctures, primarily because no water must be allowed in or near them. Introducing water into a medicinal oil at any stage will quickly encourage spoiling. Oils' shelf life is also shorter than tinctures'; you can generally expect your herbal oils to last six to twelve months, after which time they may become "flat" or rancid. Use oils as topical remedies for a variety of ailments, including sore muscles, sprains, burns, cuts, scrapes, cradle cap, dandruff, dry skin; in cosmetics; and for massage or bath applications. An herbal oil is also the first ingredient in an herbal salve, as discussed later in this chapter.

Making an Herbal Oil

An herbal oil is simply a tincture that will be used externally instead of internally and that is made with vegetable oil instead of alcohol, glycerin, or vinegar.

When making herbal oils, you can use both fresh and dried herbs, though fresh herbs produce a more robust product with a better fragrance, color, and potency. But don't make them too fresh: always wilt your leaves and flowers for a few hours before chopping them. This allows excess moisture to evaporate; too much moisture will spoil the oil.

Ensure that all your pots, pans, spoons, measuring cups, and so on are completely dry before making your oil.

SIMPLER'S METHOD

To make the oil, gather dried or harvest fresh leaves or flowers on a dry day after all dew has evaporated. If it's a cloudy day or has been raining, wait for a sunny day to harvest your oil herbs.

Spread the fresh herbs out on a screen or newspaper to wilt. Make sure they are in a single layer and no leaves cover each other. Allow them to wilt for several hours or overnight.

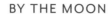

BY THE MOON

Lunar activity has always affected human cycles as well as more obvious cycles such as ocean tides. Midwives and obstetricians have long noticed that more babies are born on full moons, and people generally feel more sociable and willing to go out on a full moon. More parties take place and more crimes are committed on full moons. Likewise, plants feel lunar effects and respond accordingly, as sap and phytochemicals rise to the surface. It's as if everything is being drawn from the earth and pulled upward. For this reason, many herbalists harvest aboveground plant parts (leaves, berries, and flowers) on full moons and belowground roots on new moons when the earth's pull is greater. I tend to decant tinctures on a full moon, when it seems plant energies are ready to "get out."

Chop them thoroughly with a knife to get the most surface area. Do *not* chop them in a blender; this introduces too much air and releases too much water from the plant, which can cause spoilage. Place the herb(s) in a clean, dry, 1-quart glass jar. Pack the jar tight and nearly full if you are using fresh herbs; if you're using dried, pack the jar half-full.

Prepare the menstruum (liquid). Use oil(s) that you would feel comfortable putting on your body. Think about the final product: will it simply be an oil, or will you combine it with wax to make a salve? If the final product will be an oil, then thin oils such as sunflower, sweet almond, safflower, and grapeseed are acceptable. If the final product will be a salve, then thicker oils such as canola, olive, jojoba, and coconut are better choices.

Pour the oil(s) into the 1-quart jar using a long, thin stick, a wooden-handled spoon, or a skewer to poke around the sides to release air bubbles.

(Make sure *no* water gets into the jar!) Fill to within ¼ inch of the rim of the jar. Clean the rim and cap the jar tightly.

Label it in two locations. On two pieces of masking tape write the name of the herb(s), the date, and the menstruum used. Place one piece of tape on the lid and one on the side of the jar. Place the jar in a cool, dark cabinet on top of a plate. This is important, because the oil can ooze up out of the cap and ruin counters, cabinets, and shelves. Shake the jar daily for two to four weeks.

Decant (strain) the liquid and press the herbs firmly to get out as much valuable liquid as possible. Compost the leftover herbs. Bottle the oil; label it; and store it in a cool, dark cabinet.

It will have a shelf life of approximately six to twelve months.

QUICK METHOD

To make the oil, gather dried or harvest fresh leaves or flowers on a dry day after all dew has evaporated. If it's a cloudy day or it has been raining, wait for a sunny day to harvest your oil herbs.

Spread the fresh herbs out on a screen or newspaper to wilt. Make sure they are in a single layer and that no leaves cover each other. Allow them to wilt for several hours or overnight.

Chop them thoroughly with a knife to get the most surface area. Do *not* chop them in a blender. Place 1 cup fresh (or ½ cup dried) herbs in a clean, dry saucepan.

Prepare the menstruum (liquid). Think about the final product: will this be an oil forever, or will you combine it with wax to make a salve? If the final product will be an oil, then thin oils such as sunflower, safflower, and grapeseed are acceptable, *but* you should use the Simpler's Method described above. If the final product will be a salve, then thicker oils such as canola and olive oils are better choices, and this Quick Method is acceptable.

Pour 1 cup oil into the saucepan and stir it into the herbs. Gently heat the mixture on low heat for 20 to 30 minutes, making sure the oil never bubbles or boils. (You don't want crispy fried herbs!) You just want to let the heat suggest to the herbs that they release their goodness.

Decant (strain) the liquid and press the herbs firmly to get out as much valuable liquid as possible, being careful not to burn yourself. Compost the leftover herbs. Bottle the oil; label it; and store it in a cool, dark cabinet.

It will have a shelf life of approximately six to twelve months.

Making an Herbal Salve

A medicinal salve, or ointment, is an herb-infused oil that has been combined with a thick fat, which in the past was animal fat (rendered lard), vegetable shortening, or beeswax. Salves offer a wealth of functions and are essential to any medicine cabinet or first-aid kit. Use salves topically to treat cuts, scrapes, wounds, and burns, or as bug repellent, lotions, lip balm, and more. The choice of herbs and essential oils makes for different medicines and uses.

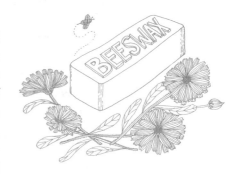

When making herbal salves, be sure to use dedicated equipment, as noted earlier in the chapter. Choose a stainless steel or enamel saucepan that will be used only for making salves, as the beeswax will never completely come out of it. Also use utensils such as cutting boards, knives, and measuring cups that you use only with beeswax. This will save many a headache in the future!

Use either of the methods described in the last section to make an herbal oil. Instead of bottling the oil after straining the herbs out, pour it into a dry glass measuring cup. Measure the oil, then pour it into a clean, dry saucepan.

Chop the beeswax. This can be purchased as "beads" at health food stores, but it is much better in chunks or blocks. Look for wax that has not been bleached or filtered; chemicals are often used to bleach wax or make it more salable. Wax straight from the beehive is best. (See the Resources section at the end of the book for beeswax suppliers.) Do not use paraffin or candle wax; these will ruin your salve. Chop or shave your beeswax into $1/4$ to $1/2$-inch slivers or chunks.

In a dry measuring cup, measure $1/4$ cup wax chunks for every 1 cup oil. For example, if you poured 1 cup oil into the saucepan, use $1/4$ cup wax.

Drop the wax into the saucepan with oil and heat them gently. As the wax melts, you may stir in essential oils if desired. For every 1 cup of oil, 5 to 10 drops of essential oil may be sufficient.

Once the wax is completely melted, quickly pour the solution from the pan into a pouring container such as a (dedicated) clean glass measuring cup. Pour the salve from this into individual glass or ceramic containers.

Add more essential oil if desired and cap the containers tightly. Allow the salve to cool. Don't move the containers for at least an hour; they'll cool from the bottom up and the color will lighten to a pale shade. Label the containers and store them in a cool, dry cabinet.

The salve will have a shelf life of approximately eighteen to twenty-four months.

WHAT YOU DON'T WANT

As an herbal crafter, you may happily avoid unnecessary and potentially harmful chemicals that many commercial skin and beauty products contain. A quick look at a few labels of "natural" body care products reveal these barely pronounceable ingredients: Phynoxyethanol, Imidazolidinyl Urea, Butyl Methoxydibenzoylmethane, Methylparaben, Acrylates/C10-C30, Alkyl Acrylate Crosspolymer, Butylene/Ethylene/Styrene Copolymer, Disodium EDTA, DMDM Hydantoin, Yellow 5 (C1 19140), Yellow 6 (C1 15985) . . .

Body Lotions (Creams)

Intimidated at the thought of making lotions and face creams? Me too. For years I've experimented with various lotion and cream recipes that turned out greasy or separated. Trickier than salves, which are fairly basic, lotions can be daunting because the primary ingredients—oils and water— don't naturally mix. Lotions tend to separate, and once they do, they spoil quickly.

I finally cobbled together a basic recipe for a thick "lotion" that's spreadable and rich, deeply penetrating, and beautiful in a jar. Best as an all-over body moisturizer (it's fantastic after sun exposure), it also makes a hydrating nighttime face cream. I find it's best applied sparingly at night so that the oils can penetrate; it goes on slightly greasy and shiny but penetrates quickly, bestowing a radiant and smooth complexion. In the morning, the skin is smooth, clear, and supple. Refrigerate this cream so it will last up to a month; otherwise, it has a shelf life of approximately five to seven days.

This formula blends one part oil to one part water. It is simple and easy, yielding three 2-ounce jars of lotion while using minimal ingredients. This small yield allows you to experiment freely with the recipe without worrying about using a lot of costly supplies. When you're satisfied with the process, move on to more complex formulas.

¼ cup water (or flower hydrosol, such as rose or lavender)
¼ cup aloe vera juice
¼ cup coconut oil (the solidified kind in a tub)
¼ cup sweet almond oil (or jojoba oil, which turns the cream a light
    yellow)
Essential oil of your choice (optional)

Combine the water and aloe vera juice in a small glass bowl. Set the mixture aside.

Heat the coconut oil gently until it's clear, about 3 minutes. With a spatula, slide the coconut oil into a large bowl or glass measuring cup. Add the sweet almond or jojoba oil.

While whisking with one hand or blending with an electric mixer, slowly pour the water-aloe mixture into the oils. Whisk quickly. The mixture will become white and thick.

At this point, add 2 to 4 drops of essential oil for fragrance and as a natural preservative if desired.

Pour the finished cream into three jars, cap them tightly, and label them. Store the cream in the refrigerator.

It will have a shelf life of up to one month in the refrigerator.

Water-Based Medicines

Water-based remedies are probably among the oldest medicines in the world. Few things are simpler than steeping herbs in water, either over heat or in a simple glass jar in the sunlight. Water remedies are my favorite because of their simplicity—teas are easily ingested and they help hydrate the body, as well. Water-based remedies are like vitamins in that they are quickly absorbed by the body and just as quickly eliminated.

When making herbal tea blends, combine the dried herbs in a glass jar with a tight lid or in a tightly sealed, food-grade plastic bag, and from this supply you can measure out what you need to make your tea. Store this jar or bag in a dry, dark pantry or cabinet.

The water-based beverages we use for medicine have earned various names, including *teas*, *tisanes*, *infusions*, *decoctions*, and *standard brews*, though most people simply say *tea*. Here are the distinctions and how to make them.

Making Black, Green, and Other Caffeinated Teas

True tea is brewed from the leaves of the *Camellia sinensis*, a small tree typically grown in China. The astringent leaves contain tannins and caffeine, and depending on how they are processed and fermented, they will produce robustly flavored black tea, bitter green tea, or mellow white teas or oolongs.

To make a cup of black tea, pour 1 cup boiling water over 1 teaspoon dried tea leaves and steep between 3 and 8 minutes, keeping in mind that the longer the tea brews, the more bitter it will taste. Sweeten as desired. The addition of milk will counteract the tannins, keeping the tea from upsetting the stomach.

Making an Herbal Tea or Tisane

A tea or tisane is simply an herbal beverage that is made from plants other than the true tea plant. Though the herbs in an herbal tea or tisane can be steeped for any length of time, most teas or tisanes are light in color, fragrant, and gentle, while infusions (see below, "Making an Herbal Infusion") are dark in color and strongly medicinal. Don't let the terminology confuse you: it's really just about how long the herbs are steeped in the water, because the longer they steep, the more minerals, vitamins, tannins, essential oils, and other chemicals they release into the liquid.

Herbal tea that is brewed briefly—say, 2 to 12 minutes—makes a lightly flavored, delicious, and gently healing beverage. Sometimes we want to brew herbs overnight to extract as many minerals as possible; this is called an infusion. Don't worry about whether you're making a tisane, tea, or infusion, since the terminology is not as important as the process. Practice and experimentation will reveal how long each plant needs to steep to make a tasty beverage for pleasure or a healing beverage for medicine.

Every herb will be prepared differently, which is part of the learning process for new herbalists. The list below is an introductory guideline to determine how long to steep particular herbs for gentle healing teas or tisanes. Bitter herbs require a shorter brewing time of 2 to 4 minutes, while mild or delicate herbs and flowers need a longer brewing time of 9 to 12 minutes. For example, since motherwort contains strong bitter principles and quickly creates a very bitter beverage, it needs to steep only for a brief time, about 2 to 4 minutes. (I often brew other herbs for a long time and add the bitter motherwort at the very end.) Lemon balm, however, is not bitter and takes a while to release its citrus flavor, so steeping it for 9 to 12 minutes or even for several hours is appropriate. Use your best judgment and experiment with taste, fragrance, and color. Sweeten your teas with honey, stevia leaf, or maple syrup.

To make a cup of tea, place 1 to 2 teaspoons of dried herb into a metal tea infuser or a glass or enamel teapot. Pour 1 cup boiling water over this and steep according to the guidelines below. Strain, sweeten, and drink hot; alternatively, chill and drink iced.

Suggested Brewing Times for Delicious Teas

Light brew (2–4 minutes)
Dandelion leaf
Motherwort
Green and black teas
Calendula flower
Dong quai
Elder flower

Medium brew (5–8 minutes)
Violet leaf
Peppermint/spearmint
Catnip
Nettle
Rose petals
Oatstraw
Holy basil
Self-heal
Chamomile

Long brew (9-12 minutes)
Red clover
Lemon balm
Lemon verbena
Violet flower
Dandelion root
Rose hips
Ginger root

Making an Herbal Infusion

An *infusion* is a water-based medicine in which an herb's softer aerial parts (leaves and flowers) have been infused or "steeped" in just-boiled water for a length of time sufficient to extract medicinal properties and minerals. Gypsy herbalist Juliette de Bairacli Levy coined the term *standard brew*, and Susun Weed revised it to *infusion* to indicate that the herbs have steeped much longer than in a simple tea or tisane.

Infusions are a very effective form of botanical medicine, especially for long-term, chronic conditions. They are also the basis for other water-based medicines, such as syrups and compresses (see below, "Making a Syrup" and "Making a Compress"). Pouring boiling water over dried herbs bursts the plants' cell walls, releasing beneficial nutrients including vitamins, minerals, essential oils, and tannins into the tea where they can be easily digested and absorbed into the bloodstream. It tends to be easier to burst the walls of dried plants than fresh plants, but if you're using fresh herbs, simply triple the quantity and chop them finely with a knife. An infusion is considered medicinal strength and can be given to children and adults following the dosage guidelines on pages 287–90.

Since you'll normally drink between 2 and 4 cups per day, it's impractical to make infusions by the cup; instead, make them by the quart and drink the entire quart throughout the day. Any leftover tea can be refrigerated and should be consumed the following day or poured onto plants as fertilizer.

To make an infusion, place 1 ounce (approximately 1 to 2 cups) of dried herb in a stainless steel, glass, or enamel pot. Cover the herb with 1 quart fresh boiling water and cover tightly. Steep 15 to 20 minutes or up to 4 hours for gentle infusions, or overnight for strong infusions. Keep in mind that the longer some herbs steep, the more bitter the infusion can taste. Ideal herbs for overnight infusions include nettle, oatstraw, alfalfa, red clover, lemon balm, violet, lemon verbena, cleavers, raspberry, and self-heal.

Alternatively, make an infusion by placing 1 ounce (approximately 1 to 2 cups) of dried herb in a pot on the stove and covering the herb with 1 quart cold water. Bring this very slowly to a boil, covered, and remove from heat. Allow this to sit undisturbed for 15 to 20 minutes or up to 4 hours for gentle infusions or overnight for strong infusions.

Strain, reserving as much liquid as possible and composting the leftover herbs.

To sweeten the infusion, gently reheat it and add honey, stevia, or maple syrup; ¼ to 1 teaspoon honey is usually sufficient for 1 cup of infusion. Experiment with sweeteners; stevia is a lovely plant with naturally sweet leaves that you can crumble into your teapot or steep along with the tea, and licorice can be brewed with other herbs to release its natural sweetness.

Store a hot infusion in a thermos, or a cold infusion in the refrigerator. Drink 2 to 4 cups daily for most tonic infusions (or follow the individual recipe recommendations and the dosage guidelines on pages 287–90. Be sure to drink all of the infusion within one 24-hour period, or refrigerate leftover tea and drink within 24 hours. As water-based remedies, teas lose their potency quickly and do not keep. If you're taking herbal infusions regularly, make a habit of steeping your herbs each evening.

Note: When drinking teas and infusions, the temperature of the liquid can affect how the herb acts in your body. For example, yarrow (*Achillea millefolium*), a wonderful herb for colds and flu, will make you sweat if it is taken as a hot infusion. This is called a diaphoretic and it's an effective way to lower a fever. However, if you drink yarrow tea cold, it will act as a diuretic and send you to the bathroom. This is useful for relieving the body of excess fluid and increasing blood flow through the kidneys. Generally, though, especially for colds and flu, take teas as hot as possible without burning the mouth.

Making an Herbal Decoction

A *decoction* is a liquid medicine that has cooked on the stovetop. It consists of the harder and woodier parts of plants such as roots, bark, seeds, and tough stems.

To make an herbal decoction, select and gather the seeds and roots you wish to use. Wash and chop them with a knife, then place them in a deep teapot or soup pot. Cover them with fresh cold water. For each ounce of fresh roots, use 1 quart water; for each 1 to 2 teaspoons of dried roots, use 1 cup water. Allow the mixture to sit for 1 to 2 hours.

Turn on the heat and slowly bring the water to a boil; immediately reduce to a simmer and cover the pot tightly. Allow it to simmer on low heat from 20 minutes to 3 hours.

Remove the pot from the heat. Allow it to sit, still covered, overnight.

Strain the herbs, reserving as much liquid as possible. Compost the remaining herbs.

If you wish to sweeten the decoction, gently reheat it and add honey or a sweetener of your choice; $\frac{1}{2}$ to 1 teaspoon honey is usually sufficient for 1 cup of decoction.

Store a warm decoction in a thermos and a cold decoction in the refrigerator. Drink at least three cups daily for most tonic infusions (or follow the individual recipe recommendations and dosage guidelines on pages 287–90). Drink your decoction within 24 hours; since it has no preservatives, it will not keep. If you're drinking decoctions regularly, establish a habit of steeping the herbs each evening.

Making a Syrup

A *syrup* is a thick, sweetened infusion or decoction. Usually pleasant tasting, it is a great way to mask more unpleasant tasting herbs and bitters, as well as coax a child into taking his or her medicine. Syrups are my favorite sweeteners for teas; simply use them in place of sugar or honey. They are easy to make but must be stored in the refrigerator.

To make a syrup, gather dried or harvest fresh herbs; you can use the leaves, flowers, buds, seeds, or bark, depending on the plant. If you're using fresh herbs, clean and chop them with a knife. Prepare 3 cups fresh herbs or 1 cup dried.

Place the herbs in a pot and cover them with 3 cups cold, fresh water. Bring the mixture to a boil, then gently simmer, covered loosely so steam may escape. Simmer it 2 to 4 hours or until the liquid has reduced by two-thirds.

Strain the herbs and measure the remaining liquid. You should have roughly 1 cup. Return the liquid to the pot and add ½ to ¾ cup honey, maple syrup, or sugar. Gently heat the syrup until all ingredients are completely blended, about 3 to 5 minutes.

Pour the syrup into a glass jar, cap it tightly, and label it. Store it in the refrigerator.

It will have a shelf life of approximately three to six months in the refrigerator.

Making a Compress (Fomentation)

A *compress*, also called a *fomentation*, is the external application of a warm, concentrated herbal infusion. It is like a poultice, but instead of applying the leaves directly to the wound, the leaves are removed from the liquid and the infusion (tea) is applied directly to the wound with a soft cloth. This method is preferable for treating children and for messy wounds where it would be inadvisable to lay bits of leaves on top. A compress is more elegant, cleaner, and more familiar, as it appears to be a big bandage.

It's also safer for use around the eyes, on burns, and with open or bleeding wounds. You can use either fresh or dried plant material.

Good easy-to-gather herbs for a compress include mint, plantain, yarrow, rosemary, oregano, lemon balm, pine/hemlock tips, and oak bark or leaves.

To make a compress, gather dried or harvest fresh herbs. If you're using fresh herbs, clean and chop them with a knife; you will need approximately 3 cups. If you're using dried herbs, you will need 1 cup. Place the herbs in a shallow pan.

Pour 3 cups fresh cold water over the herbs and bring the mixture to a boil. Immediately reduce the heat, cover the pot, and simmer on low heat for about 15 minutes until the liquid is dark and fragrant. The water is now an infusion full of the plant's properties.

Prepare two or three clean cloths. These are best when made of cotton or flannel, but they can be handkerchiefs, bandanas, or some other cloth in an emergency situation or while camping.

Strain the herbs, reserving as much liquid as possible, and return the liquid to the pan. Place the cloths in the water and allow them to soak up the "tea."

Pull one cloth from the pan and wring it lightly; you want a lot of tea in the cloth but not so much that it drips everywhere. This cloth is your compress. Gently apply the warm compress to the wound and wrap it loosely with a dry cloth. Allow it to remain in direct contact with the skin until the heat is gone, then remove it and apply more infusion with a second cloth. Repeat this process for 20 to 30 minutes, then discard any unused liquid.

Making a Poultice

A *poultice* is the external application of warm, wet, macerated herbs. These herbs are generally of the wound-healing (vulnerary) variety, such as yarrow, elder, red clover, or plantain. (Use care with herbs such as comfrey and mullein, as they have tiny hairs that may irritate a fresh wound.) The fresh leaves are pounded or macerated just to the point where the natural juices flow and the leaves become supple. These leaves are then placed directly on the wound so the juices smother it and healing can begin. This can be a messy process and is certainly not elegant, but it's effective and is a wonderful use of fresh herbs.

To make a poultice, choose and harvest your herbs, clean, and chop them with a knife. Place approximately 2 to 3 cups chopped herbs in a shallow pan.

Pour 1 cup cold fresh water over the herbs and bring them to a simmer. The herbs should be warm, and there should be just enough water to cover them. The goal is to tenderize the leaves so they can be placed comfortably on the wound.

When the leaves are supple, wet, warm, and pliable, carefully withdraw a small handful from the pan and lay them on top of the wounded skin. If there is pain, burning, or prickling, remove the herbs and place a thin layer of muslin or cotton on the skin. Wrap the herbs in a covering layer of muslin, cotton flannel, or plastic wrap, and allow them to rest on the wound until the heat is gone. Remove the poultice and reapply with fresh herbs. Encourage the patient to relax and drink healing teas while resting under the poultice. (The practice of poulticing is also used to draw objects such as cysts, tumors, and splinters from the body.)

Making a Plaster

Similar to a poultice, a *plaster* involves powdered herbs that are mixed with warm water and applied directly to the skin or over a thin piece of gauze. Mustard is often used because it is easily available as a powder and is warming and stimulating, but other herbs—including powdered ginger, powdered yarrow, and even powdered rose petals—can work well for various situations.

To make a plaster, mix 2 tablespoons powdered mustard seed or powdered ginger with 2 tablespoons wheat flour or cornmeal. (This dilutes the potency of the herb, which can burn skin at full strength.) If using yarrow or rose, use 4 tablespoons of the herb or dilute it with only 1 tablespoon of flour, as these herbs are not burning.

Mix in 2 to 6 tablespoons warm (not boiling) water until the mixture has a thick, spreadable paste consistency.

Gently place a thin piece of gauze or cotton cloth on the skin. Spread the paste on the gauze. Leave the poultice on as long as possible, from 8 to 30 minutes. Rest and repeat every 30 minutes until all plaster is used. Store the powdered herb in a tightly sealed container for the next use; it will remain potent for approximately one year.

Making a Hydrosol

Another water medicine that uses fresh herbs, a hydrosol is a lovely preparation with a long history. First discovered thousands of years ago, distilled plant waters and essential oils were popular with ladies of old as hair rinses, skin treatments, and even flavorings.

You will require a distiller to make true hydrosols (flower waters) and to extract a plant's essential oils. It takes a great deal of plant matter to isolate even an ounce of essential oil, which is why these oils can be quite expensive. If you are lucky enough to own a distiller, follow the manufacturer's directions and either refrigerate the final product or add witch hazel as a preservative. Flower water—the "by-product" of essential oil extraction—is more abundant and less expensive, and (depending on the plant used) it can be taken internally, used in cooking, or applied externally, often to the face or chilled and sprayed on the skin to refresh it.

If you don't have a distiller, simply purchase the following ingredients and combine them to your liking. This makes for a lovely spritzer to be sprayed on the face (eyes closed), the skin, and even pillows and linens for a soothing (or tantalizing) fragrance. Stored in the fridge, it is a wonderful pick-me-up on hot summer days.

Choose your essential oils. Soothing scents include rose, sandalwood, patchouli, lavender, Peru balsam, violet, and chamomile. Stimulating and invigorating scents include catnip, yarrow, Queen Anne's lace, lemon, lemongrass, peppermint, and rosemary. A little essential oil goes a long way, so purchase it by the ¼ ounce.

To make a hydrosol, combine ¾ cup distilled water with ¼ cup distilled witch hazel (from the pharmacy). Add 5 to 15 drops of the essential oil and pour the mixture into a container with a spray nozzle.

Alternatively, to make four 2-ounce spritzer bottles, combine ¾ cup distilled water with ¼ cup distilled witch hazel. Pour the mixture into the four bottles. Add 5 drops of essential oil to each bottle. This allows you to use different scents and create up to four different spritzers.

The hydrosol will have a shelf life of approximately twelve months.

Honey-Based Medicines

Honey is naturally medicinal and lauded for both its external use as a dressing for wounds and topical ulcers and its internal use to address sore throats and coughs. Honey medicines are among the easiest and most pleasant remedies to make—and take! (Instructions for making herbal syrups with honey, maple syrup, or sugar are given in the above section "Making a Syrup.")

Making an Oxymel

Ancient apothecaries used the term *oxymel* to refer to a honey-based syrup preserved with vinegar or a vinegar tincture sweetened with honey; either way, it's a delicious blend of sugar and acid that's easy to prepare. Often used to disguise foul-tasting herbal concoctions, an elixir can also be a tasty medicine, especially when using tart or tangy herbs such as lemon balm, fennel, or rose hips. Tart, tangy, sweet-and-sour—delicious!

Start by making a vinegar tincture following the steps described earlier in this chapter.

To 1 cup prepared vinegar tincture, add ¾ cup honey. Gently heat the mixture in a small saucepan until blended.

Bottle the elixir, label it, and store it in the pantry. Don't put it in the refrigerator, because the honey will lose its liquidity. Take 1 teaspoon 2 to 3 times daily.

The elixir will have a shelf life of approximately twelve months.

Making an Herbal Honey

This is by far my favorite way to use herbs. Honeys are beyond easy, and the result is so delicious, it just can't be believed. Slather your toast with it, and stir it into teas. (Or follow my husband's lead and just eat it straight from the jar with a spoon.)

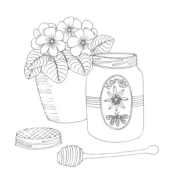

To make an herbal honey, harvest fresh herbs. (Don't use dried plant material for this preparation; the best results are only from fresh plants.) Leaves and flowers work best, especially lavender and mint. Chop them roughly with a knife immediately before you add the honey.

Place the herbs in a casserole or bowl, and pour the honey over them. Generally, for every 2 to 3 cups of herbs, you'll need 6 cups of honey. Cover the casserole and allow the mixture to steep overnight.

Place the casserole over low heat and gently warm the honey until it is clear and runny. Quickly strain it into jars. You can add a drop or two of essential oil if you wish, but I find it unnecessary. The honey will be extremely fragrant and taste strongly of the herb you used.

Cap the jars, label them, and store them at room temperature.

The honey will have a shelf life of approximately twelve months.

Powdered Herbal Medicines

Powdered herbal medicines are a great way to incorporate dried herbs into your herbal repertoire. Dried and powdered herbs are convenient, easy to take, and in some ways more palatable.

You can purchase ready-made powders at reputable sources (see the Resources section at the end of this book) or make your own powders. To do so, harvest your chosen herbs and carefully dry them on a screen or newspaper in the shade, one layer deep and with no leaves covering each other, until crisp. Crush them with a mortar and pestle, or grind them in a dedicated coffee or spice grinder. Sieve the herbs through a strainer to remove any large pieces. Store them in a labeled freezer bag or a glass jar with a tight-fitting lid.

Making Capsules

Capsules are popular because they conveniently deliver bitter or unpleasant-tasting herbs, such as goldenseal or garlic, to the digestive tract. Powdered herbs can be blended, measured, and placed into gelatin or vegan capsules to be swallowed, requiring no brewing of tea or chewing of tablets. Most health food stores stock two types of capsule: the gelatin capsule, which is made from animal collagen, and the vegan (or cellulose) capsule, which is made from the starchy cellulose of pine or poplar trees. When purchasing capsules, be sure to identify its size: the small "0" size capsule holds between 150 and 300 milligrams of herbal powder and is most easily swallowed by children, while the larger "00" capsules hold between 250 and 500 milli-grams and are more suitable for adults. Filling the capsules with powder can be tricky, though there are a few rudimentary "machines" on the market for about $30 with which you can fill between 24 and 100 capsules at once. In my experience, it takes less than ½ cup of herbal powder to fill 100 capsules, but it is tedious work that can take up to an hour. However, encapsulating your own herbal powders guarantees you are ingesting no excipients, bind-ers, fillers, or preservatives in the medicine itself, as in commercial capsules. See the Resources section at the end of this book for retailers of capsules and filling machines.

Making a Suppository

A *suppository*, or *bolus*, is one of those delightful ancient herbal terms for a common treatment—an herbal preparation that is inserted into a body cavity (usually the vagina or rectum) to introduce needed medicine right where it will do the most good. (In other words, it's not digested or applied externally. It's "orificial.") You can use this type of preparation for treating yeast infections, prostate inflammation, hemorrhoids, and cervical dysplasia.

To make a suppository, gather together aluminum foil, thick magic markers or pencils, a glass measuring cup, a double boiler, cocoa butter or coconut oil, and the powdered herbs of your choice.

Wrap the aluminum foil around a marker or pencil and tighwtly crimp one end closed, leaving the other open. Remove the marker and stand this first mold upright in a glass measuring cup while you make the others (a supply of six to seven is usually advisable for common problems).

In a double boiler, gently and slowly heat 1 cup cocoa butter or coconut oil for 1 minute until it has liquefied.

Mix in 1 to 4 teaspoons of the powdered herbs, stirring constantly. Remove from heat.

Pour the liquid into your ready-made, room-temperature aluminum-foil molds; crimp the open ends shut; and place them in a small dish in the freezer.

Take them out after 10 to 15 minutes, remove the foil, and slice the suppositories on a cutting board to the desired length. With your fingers, quickly smooth the edges if desired and rewrap each suppository. Store in the refrigerator (labeled!) and insert one each night upon retiring. Wear a pad or pantiliner in your underwear to catch leaks.

The suppositories will have a shelf life of approximately two months in the refrigerator.

Making Body Powder

Body powders wick sweat and moisture away from the skin, which can be cooling and satisfying on a hot summer day. Many commercial powders include talc, which can cause serious problems when inhaled or applied to the skin. The herbal powders I describe use arrowroot, a naturally starchy root that, when dried and powdered, makes a lovely body dust. Natural clays have also been used the world over for absorbing moisture and drying the skin. You can scent the powders as you desire.

In a dry bowl, combine 1 cup arrowroot powder, 1 cup white kaolin clay, and $1/2$ cup powdered rose petals (or another scented herb of your choice, such as violet flowers, lemongrass, and so on). If desired, you can add 5 to 10 drops of essential oil, which will readily absorb and not affect the consistency of the powder. Stir the mixture gently with a stainless steel spoon.

Gently spoon the powder into containers with sifter lids, such as spice jars. This powder will keep indefinitely.

Astringent Herbal Medicines

Distilled witch hazel is readily available in pharmacies across the country. It is a colorless, odorless liquid distilled from the twigs, branches, and bark of the witch hazel tree (*Hamamelis virginiana*). The bottles of witch hazel you'll find at most pharmacies include 14 percent isopropyl alcohol as a preservative, and they must only be used externally, since they are toxic if taken internally. Because it is naturally astringent, witch hazel quickly absorbs chemicals from other plants and makes a wonderful menstruum for a variety of herbs; it is also an ideal ingredient for facial astringents and wound remedies.

Making a Liniment

A *liniment* is an old-fashioned but effective remedy. Made in much the same way as a tincture, a liniment is a liquid concentrate of herbs that can be applied to the skin with a cotton ball, a cloth, or the fingers. Most liniments relieve sore joints, inflamed muscles, arthritis, and rheumatic pain. They are made with either rubbing alcohol or witch hazel, and *you must never ingest them*—they are for *external use only*! Keep them away from children.

To make a liniment, gather dried or harvest fresh herbs. If you are using fresh herbs, clean and chop them with a knife. Herbs that are useful for sore joints and inflammation include arnica, wintergreen leaves and berries, meadowsweet leaves, white willow inner bark, Saint-John's-wort, rosemary, elder leaves, comfrey, and peppermint.

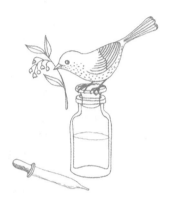

Place the herb(s) in a clean, dry, 1-pint glass jar. Pack the jar tight and nearly full if you are using fresh herbs; if you're using dried, pack the jar half-full. Pour 2 cups rubbing (isopropyl) alcohol or distilled witch hazel over the herbs and use a long, thin stick, a wooden-handled spoon, or a skewer to poke around the sides to release air bubbles.

Cap the jar, label it, and allow it to sit in a cool, dark cabinet for two weeks.

Decant (strain) the liquid into a clean container and press the herbs firmly to release as much valuable liquid as possible. Compost the leftover herbs. Bottle the liniment, being sure to write "for external use only" prominently on the label. Store the bottle in a high cabinet out of children's reach.

The liniment will have a shelf life of approximately two to three years.

Making a Facial Astringent

This lovely facial wash is intended to be applied to a just-cleaned face with a cotton ball. Allow it to remain on the skin only a few moments, then apply a moisturizer such as the Red Clover Whipped Lotion in chapter 17: Beauty, Skin, and Body Care.

USING ESSENTIAL OILS

All plants have special, or active, principles that can be extracted. That's what our medicines are. One extracted principle is the *essential oil,* which is a highly concentrated, volatile oil that usually smells strong and is often antibiotic, antimicrobial, antiviral, antifungal, and so on. The distillation process pulls these volatile oils out with the evaporating water, and the oil can be skimmed off. It is sold commercially in tiny bottles—usually of one ounce or less. A few drops are all you need in most recipes in this book. As with most extracted principles, you don't want to consume essential oils alone internally. You may dilute them and use them on your skin or place them on a hot light bulb to evaporate and release their scent. Use caution in storing these oils, and keep them out of children's reach; also be wary of using certain essential oils—such as cinnamon or wintergreen—on the skin even when they are diluted, as some people may experience burning or rashes.

Though they are useful, essential oils are precious, and even rare. It takes tens of thousands of rose petals, for example, to yield less than an ounce of essential oil. This product (called rose attar) is extremely expensive, costing hundreds of dollars per half-ounce, and true attars are very difficult to obtain. A well-stocked pantry of oils for the beginning herbalist should include lemon exract/essential oil, rosemary, peppermint, lavender, clove, and something exotic and sensual such as Peru balsam or patchouli. As always, use respect and common sense when using these highly concentrated extracts on your skin.

Mixing essential oils to create a scent is a fun skill-building exercise; follow the guidelines often given for perfume making, whereby dusky base scents are mixed with lighter or sweet scents to reach a balance. Both scents will be appreciated without one being overwhelming. The best way to experiment is with a mild oil such as sunflower or safflower; get several friends together to create simple massage oils and have lots of small bottles ready. Mix and match using only a few drops of each, making note of which base oils (those with earthy or sensual fragrances) blend well with which high-note oils (those with fruity, sweet, or "sparkly" fragrances). I've found the following combinations blend well together:

Vanilla-clove
Rosemary-clove
Peru balsam–amyris–nutmeg–vanilla
Sweet orange–vanilla

Scents such as lavender stand on their own.

To make an astringent, gather dried herbs or harvest fresh leaves or flowers (calendula, violet, and rosemary are ideal for witch hazel–based facial astringents). Chop the herbs thoroughly with a knife to get the most surface area. Do *not* chop them in a blender; this introduces too much air and releases too much water from the plant, which can cause spoilage.

Place the herb(s) in a clean, dry, 1-quart glass jar. Pack the jar tight and nearly full if you are using fresh herbs; if you're using dried, fill the jar halfway.

Pour witch hazel into the jar using a long, thin stick, a wooden-handled spoon, or a skewer to poke around the sides to release air bubbles. If only a mild or delicate astringent action is desired, fill half the jar with witch hazel and the remainder with distilled water. Fill to within ¼ inch of the rim of the jar. Clean the rim, and cap the jar tightly.

Label it in two locations. On two pieces of masking tape, write the name of the herb(s), the date, and the liquid used. Place one piece of tape on the lid and one on the side of the jar.

Place the jar in a cool, dark cabinet and shake it daily for two weeks.

Decant (strain) the liquid into a clean container and press the herbs firmly to get out as much valuable liquid as possible. Compost the leftover herbs. Bottle the astringent; label it; and store it in a cool, dark cabinet.

It will have a shelf life of approximately twelve months.

Making Bath Salts

Similar to witch hazel preparations, bath salts tone the skin with a tightening and dehydrating action, so they are included here with other astringent medicines.

Concentrated bath salts are wonderful for long hearty soaks on a cold night. They can be warming and stimulating, and they are useful during a cleanse at any time of year. Make your salts with the best-quality Dead Sea and Epsom salts you can find (see the Resources section at the end of the book). Do *not* use iodized table salt. Grocery-store Epsom salts can be procured from questionable sources (such as aluminum refineries), while better-quality salts, such as Dead Sea salts and top-quality Epsom salts, are always solar dried and often hand harvested. Remember, anything you put on your skin is absorbed into your body, so you don't want any harmful chemicals in your ingredients.

During a bath or soak with these salts, be sure to drink plenty of fresh, clean, cold water, and refrain from staying in a hot bath for too long. Experiment with water therapy by moving from a hot bath into a cool shower to stimulate your immune system.

To make bath salts, combine 1 cup Dead Sea salts, 2 cups Epsom salts, and $1/2$ cup baking soda (sodium bicarbonate) in a large, dry bowl; the bowl can be ceramic, porcelain, glass, or stainless steel but not wood. Stir the mixture well.

Gently drizzle 2 tablespoons vegetable glycerin into the dry mixture, stirring constantly and pressing out clumps.

Gently stir 10 to 15 drops of the essential oil of your choice (lavender or pure vanilla extract for soothing baths, lemon or balsam fir for stimulating, cleansing baths) into the mixture. (See the sidebar "Using Essential Oils.") The essential oils and glycerin will be absorbed quickly. Pour the salts into a sturdy glass jar and cap with a lid or cork. A layer of plastic wrap can be placed under the cork to help retain the fragrance.

The salts will last indefinitely.

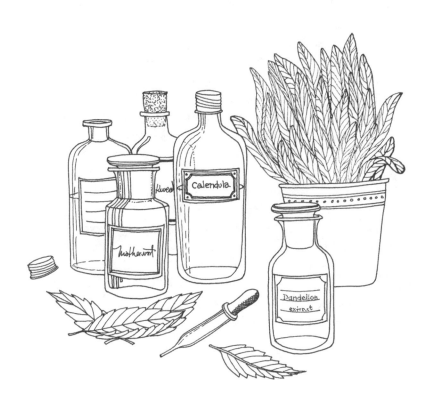

Part Three

RECIPES AND REMEDIES
FOR THE WHOLE FAMILY

Crafts make us feel rooted, give us a sense of belonging, and connect us with our history. Our ancestors used to create these crafts out of necessity, and now we do them for fun, to make money, and to express ourselves.

—Phyllis George

Chapter Five

FOR THE EXPECTANT
AND NEW MOTHER

There is nothing like the whirlwind life change of being pregnant. Whether you've planned it or not; are expecting a single, twins, or triplets; or will give birth in summer or winter—you are a creative being bringing new life into the world. It's a time of expansion, growth, learning, excitement, and bonding with a new person—though you've never met face-to-face.

Pregnancy should be approached with respect, awe, and compassion, not only toward the baby forming within your body but also toward your body itself. Nurturing your new mommy body is essential and will bring balance to a world that often focuses on the baby in the "vessel." The formulas in this chapter will nourish both your growing baby and you to help you ease into your role with grace, health, and a good dollop of humor. Protecting and nourishing your own body will naturally protect and nourish the baby within; your strength, fitness, and health will be your baby's first gifts.

CALCIUM

Many women make it through pregnancy without experiencing calcium loss. But some expectant mothers' bodies become calcium donation centers, providing the growing baby with bones and teeth through constant and repeated withdrawals. It's difficult to put the calcium back, and some women suffer as a result. I knew one woman who lost three teeth during pregnancy; they simply fell out. Other women may realize the effects of calcium depletion in their menopausal years, when osteoporosis sets in. But calcium protects not just bones and teeth; it is essential for muscle control, nerve function, proper glandular secretion, and blood clotting.

If you need to enhance calcium intake and absorption, add the following simple brews and foods to your diet. Eat dairy products (especially yogurt), meat as desired, some seafood (especially oysters and sardines), and lots of beet greens and beans. Calcium is best absorbed along with sufficient vitamin D (sunlight exposure and vitamin D-fortified milk are best) and vitamin C. Avoid sodas when you're eating calcium-rich foods; the phosphorus that contributes to the carbonation can interfere with calcium absorption.

Sweet Raspberry Calcium Brew

Yields 1 quart

1 tablespoon fennel seeds

1 tablespoon poppy seeds

2 tablespoons dried red
    raspberry leaves

1 tablespoon dried nettle
    leaves

Honey

This flavorful infusion is high in calcium and can also be used to counter nausea.

Lightly crush the seeds in a mortar and pestle or a seed or coffee grinder dedicated to herbs. Combine the herbs and seeds in a 1-quart glass jar. Pour enough boiling water over them to fill the jar. Steep for 5 to 8 minutes, strain the liquid, and add honey to taste. Drink this preparation freely.

Savory Calcium Mixture

This flavorful mixture of dried herbs and seeds is high in calcium. It makes a welcome change from sweet snacks, especially during pregnancy when many women can't tolerate sweets.

Lightly toast the sesame seeds in a dry skillet on the stovetop or in a shallow pan in the oven for 3 to 4 minutes. Combine all the ingredients and store in a jar with a tight-fitting lid. There are many ways to use this herbal mixture; here are some ideas.

Yields about 1 cup

1 tablespoon sesame seeds
1 tablespoon celery seeds
1 tablespoon dill seeds
1 tablespoon fennel seeds
1 tablespoon dried savory
1 teaspoon dried oregano
Pinch salt

As a Warming Tea

This tea is comforting in winter, is high in calcium, and can be consumed when you're breast-feeding. (*Note:* Don't use parsley while breast-feeding, as it can dry up your milk supply.) Use 1 to 3 teaspoons of the herb blend per 1 cup of boiling water, steep for 5 minutes, and strain. Add a tiny pinch of salt if you want more of a brothlike tea.

As Soup Stock

Brew as directed for tea; you may strain out the solids or not. Add to soup stock while the vegetables are simmering.

In Scrambled Eggs

Sprinkle ½ teaspoon of the herb mixture into one serving of eggs or tofu.

On Steamed Greens

Sprinkle 1 teaspoon of the herb mixture into one serving of steamed or sautéed Swiss chard, turnip greens, collard greens, mustard greens, nettles, or lamb's quarters. Top with calcium-rich, chopped, dry or roasted walnuts. Add salt, pepper, oil, and vinegar to taste.

DELICIOUS PREGNANCY TONICS

Pregnancy is a great time to nourish your body and indulge in wonderfully healthy drinks, foods, massages, yoga, and fresh-air exercises. Instead of restricting yourself or putting yourself on a special diet, feel free to explore new foods and beverages. Listen to your body's cravings; they will naturally tell you what you need.

A tonic is a plant, drink, or food that can be taken safely over a long period of time to enhance health. Many tonics are drinks that are easily absorbed and can be enjoyed several times a day over the course of your

USING TONICS

You'll get the most out of your herbs—especially tonic herbs such as raspberry, nettle, alfalfa, red clover, linden, and lemon balm—if you steep them for several hours to make an infusion. An infusion is an extremely strong tea, a bone-strengthening brew you can sink your teeth into. Wise Woman herbalist Susun Weed popularized the idea of the infusion after her mentor, Juliette de Bairacli Levy, taught about teas as "standard brews" in her legendary gypsy books. Susun says she admired Juliette's teaching of brewing tonic herbs for long periods of time and changed the term *standard brew* to *infusion*.

The method is easy: Place 1 ounce (between 1 and 2 cups) dried herbs in a 1-quart jar, fill it with boiling water, and stir with a wooden spoon. Cap the jar tightly and let sit for at least 4 hours. This is the minimum length of time necessary for the minerals to dissolve. (Dried herbs are best for teas; the boiling water bursts the cell walls quickly and easily.) Keep in mind that the longer many herbs brew, the more bitter the tea will become.

pregnancy. Tonics are nutritious, tasty, often high in vitamins and minerals, and are generally easy to make—prepare a quart or more in the morning (or before bedtime), and store it in a thermos in winter or in the fridge in summer.

Red Raspberry Pregnancy Tonic Infusion

Red raspberry leaf is the quintessential herbal tonic for pregnancy, as it is highly nourishing and strengthening to the uterus. This tasty infusion is at once sweet and slightly astringent; it is an easy way to keep hydrated and to enjoy the healthy benefits of raspberry.

1 ounce dried raspberry
leaves, chopped (about
1 cup)
1 quart boiling water
Honey or maple syrup

As a Tea

Yields 1 quart

Place the dried leaves in a 1-quart glass jar or stainless steel/enamel pot or kettle. Pour the water over them and stir. Steep for 8 to 10 minutes for a pleasant beverage or overnight (4 hours minimum) for a strong, bone-strengthening tea. Strain the liquid. If you'd like to add honey or maple syrup (raspberry tea by itself has a tart, astringent flavor), gently reheat the infusion and blend in the sweetener to taste. Store in a thermos and drink 3 to 4 cups throughout the day.

As Ice Cubes

Yields approximately 2 ice cube trays

Prepare the Raspberry Pregnancy Tonic Infusion as directed, sweeten to taste, and refrigerate. Once it is chilled, pour the infusion into ice cube trays and freeze. During labor, have a friend, partner, or doula chip the cubes for you to suck on; alternatively, grind several cubes in a blender and pour a few tablespoons of raspberry tea over the top.

Raspberry Sparkle Beverage

Yields approximately 1½ quarts

1 quart sweetened and chilled Red Raspberry Pregnancy Tonic Infusion

1 12-ounce can cold ginger ale

1 teaspoon fresh lemon juice

This is a refreshing, cold, and sparkling summertime drink.

Stir all the ingredients together in a tea pitcher, cap it, and refrigerate. Enjoy this drink throughout the day.

Mother's Meadow Tea

Yields 1 quart

Choose 3 to 5 of the following dried herbs to make up 1 ounce (about 1 cup):

Raspberry leaves

Nettle leaves

Alfalfa leaves

Linden (lime blossom) flowers

Oatstraw milky tops

Dandelion leaves

1 quart boiling water

Honey, molasses, or maple syrup

This combination of tonic herbs is hearty, safe, nutritious, and delicious. The herbs are calming and lend a "meadow" fragrance to this soothing brew. Feel free to drink it hot or cold throughout pregnancy and while breast-feeding. Dandelion is helpful as a diuretic to relieve the body of excess water.

Place the herbs in a 1-quart glass jar. Cover them with the water, stir, and steep overnight (or for a minimum of 4 hours). Strain the liquid and gently reheat it. Add sweetener to taste. Pour into a hot thermos, and enjoy 3 to 4 cups throughout the day, preferably in a sturdy pottery mug with your feet up. Relax.

This is a nourishing, tasty tea blend that's safe for any stage of pregnancy. It has a slightly zingier flavor and can be a good pick-me-up.

Combine all the herbs in a freezer bag or in a jar with tight-fitting lid. Steep 1 teaspoon per cup of boiling water for 10 minutes for a light tea, or steep overnight for a nourishing, vitamin- and mineral-rich infusion. Strain the tea and sweeten to taste. Drink it freely.

Yields 1 quart

1 tablespoon dried red
    raspberry leaves
1 tablespoon dried lemon
    balm leaves
1 tablespoon dried
    oatstraw milky tops
1 tablespoon dried nettle
    leaves
1 teaspoon dried spearmint
    leaves
Honey, molasses, or maple
    syrup

MORNING SICKNESS

Most women suffer a few irritating symptoms during the wonderful time of pregnancy, such as bloating, weight gain, and fatigue. But surely nothing can be worse than morning sickness! There are as many folk cures to treat this malady as there are supposed causes, which include low blood sugar, low hydrochloric acid, or possible vitamin B_6 deficiency. There could be other culprits entirely.

Low blood sugar can result in queasiness and morning sickness. Upon rising in the morning, many pregnant women feel faint or need to vomit, and this often reflects the body's need for food—and quick. One method to avoid this is to get up in the middle of the night and eat something. Or have food ready on your bedside table to eat in the morning before you rise (sit up to avoid choking).

Suitable foods for the morning include plain crackers; crackers with peanut butter; tiny strips of dry, nongreasy bacon; celery with peanut butter; dried fruit; candied ginger; popcorn; dried seaweed; and toast. Yogurt is wonderful; have someone bring it from the refrigerator and eat small spoonfuls before getting up.

Pregnancy causes an enormous change in your body, so it's no wonder you are stricken with nausea and, in many cases, vomiting. I experienced mild morning sickness when pregnant with my son, but it was nothing compared to the nausea I felt with my daughter. (I lost eight pounds, regained fifteen, and gave birth to a seven-pound girl.) Sleep was the best medicine, so I quit my job and stayed in bed. If you find yourself in this position, make no apologies: both you and your growing child need all the nourishment and sleep you can get. As my friend Julie, a mother of five, says, "You only have one chance to grow a child."

Use these remedies and snacks to bring a sense of peace and normalcy to the day.

Wild Yam Infusion

Yields 2 cups

1 teaspoon dried wild yam root
1 teaspoon toasted sesame seeds
1 teaspoon dried chaste tree berries
1 sliver ginger
1 cup Red Raspberry Pregnancy Tonic Infusion (see page 91)
Honey or maple syrup

Not the orange sweet potato we eat in the fall, this yam is the famous root of the South American vine that is the source of the Pill. Wild yam balances hormonal production, tones the liver, and can be used in cases of premenstrual syndrome to great effect. During pregnancy, wild yam can be a useful remedy for nausea, and it combines well with tart-tasting dong quai (Angelica sinensis) or bland-tasting chaste tree berry (Vitex agnus-castus). Here's a savory "tea" for morning sickness.

Combine the herbs, roots, and seeds in a 1-quart glass jar. Cover them with boiling water and steep for 4 hours or overnight. Strain the liquid and dilute 1 cup of infusion with 1 cup Red Raspberry Pregnancy Tonic Infusion; sweeten if desired. If you can't tolerate anything sweet, add a pinch of salt or a squirt of tamari. Take sips every 15 minutes until the nausea is gone.

HERBS TO AVOID DURING PREGNANCY

While there are many wonderful herbs that nourish, protect, and heal during pregnancy, there are also some that should be avoided because they affect pregnancy in a number of ways. Emmenagogues can bring on the flow of menstrual blood and cause miscarriage; other herbs can be toxic to developing tissues. Vermifuges are strong purgative herbs that rid the body of worms or parasites. Some herbs promote uterine (or other muscle) contractions, and still others should be avoided at the end of pregnancy because they are astringent and will interfere with the body's new goal of producing breast milk (for a list of these herbs, see the sidebar "Herbs That Dry Up Breast Milk" later in the chapter).

Herbs to avoid during pregnancy include (but are not limited to) rue, black walnut, pennyroyal, black cohosh, blue cohosh, aloe, angelica, castor oil, celery seed (not the vegetable), cotton root, elecampane, feverfew, wild indigo, life root, parsley, mugwort, osha root, sweet flag (iris), tansy, thuja, and smartweed. *Note:* Black cohosh and blue cohosh can be useful near or at delivery.

Very sensitive women and those with a history of miscarriages may also wish to avoid catnip, ginger, motherwort, chamomile, sumac berries, rosemary, and thyme. Native American herbal science teaches that they stimulate heat in the body and increase peripheral blood circulation.

Morning Sickness Tincture

Yields 2 cups

Combine the following
   dried herbs in a 1-pint
   jar until it is half-full:
1 part chaste tree berries
1 part wild yam
1 part catnip
1 part raspberry leaves
½ cup grain alcohol (such
   as vodka or brandy)
½ cup water

This tincture is a convenient way to take herbs to allay nausea. When you're ready to take it, simply drop the dose in a cup of hot tea to evaporate the alcohol.

Follow the instructions in chapter 4: Medicine-Making Methods for making an alcohol tincture. Take ¼ teaspoon 3 to 4 times daily mixed in a bit of tea or water.

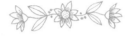

Fennel-Ginger Tea

Yields 2 cups

1 tablespoon sliced fresh
   ginger
1 tablespoon fresh or dried
   fennel seeds
2 cups boiling water
Honey or maple syrup
Lemon juice

Warming, stimulating ginger can safely be used to ease nausea, especially when sipped in small doses.

Combine the ginger and fennel, and place them in a teapot. Pour the water over the herbs and steep for 8 to 10 minutes. Strain the tea, and add honey and lemon juice to taste. Sip ¼ cup warm tea every 30 minutes until nausea subsides.

My husband loves this raw snack because it is delicious without being too sweet, and it provides enough oomph to keep him going until mealtime. It's a quick, protein-rich snack to eat when you're feeling queasy. The mixture can be rolled into balls or spread flat in a glass baking dish, chilled, and cut into squares. Keep it refrigerated.

Yields 20 to 25 bites

1 cup almond butter
½ cup raw millet
¼ cup raw sunflower or
    sesame seeds
¾ cup raisins
¼ cup maple syrup
1 tablespoon honey
½ teaspoon vanilla
¼ teaspoon cinnamon
Minced ginger candy
    (optional)
Cocoa powder,
    carob powder, or
    confectioner's sugar
    (for dusting)

Combine all the ingredients except the cocoa powder in a bowl and stir until blended. To make balls, roll 1 tablespoon in your hands or between two spoons. Lightly roll each ball in cocoa powder, carob powder, or confectioner's sugar if desired. Layer the balls between sheets of wax paper in a dish with a snap-on lid and refrigerate. Alternatively, spread the mixture in a thin layer in a 8 × 8 inch shallow glass dish and refrigerate. Slice into bars when you're ready to eat it.

This snack provides protein and calcium, and it tends to be palatable during nausea. Nibble on it when you desire something savory or substantial but can't tolerate sweets.

Yields approximately 1 cup

1 handful walnuts,
    chopped
2 tablespoons sesame
    seeds
Bland vegetable oil (such
    as canola or safflower)
Pinch salt

Lightly toast the walnuts and sesame seeds together in a dry pan over medium heat for 3 to 4 minutes, until fragrant. Remove them from the heat, and place them in a small bowl. Sprinkle with 5 to 10 drops of oil and the pinch of salt and stir to obtain a granola-like texture. Store in a tightly lidded plastic or glass container at room temperature for up to three months.

Parturition, or delivery, is the event of the baby leaving the mother's body. It's a powerful transition from pregnancy to the new experience of motherhood. You may feel extreme feelings of loss, even though you hold your beloved baby in your arms. It is more than just a physical wound or sense of loss; it can be heartbreaking to accept that you are simply no longer pregnant. Understand that for our emotional and spiritual growth, our experiences take us through cycles. Natural rhythms bring us through beginnings, middles, and invariably ends. Accepting these cycles and even appreciating the earth's wisdom in gradually guiding us through cyclical growth is the best and most nurturing way to transition into motherhood. The recipes in this section address emotional feelings of loss, the need for empowerment and strength as a new mother, and the physical wounds resulting from delivery.

New Mother's Transition Tea

Yields 1 quart

2 tablespoons dried rose petals

2 tablespoons dried lemon balm leaves

2 tablespoons dried violet flowers

½ teaspoon dried motherwort leaves

The emotionally healing herbs in this formula combine well for a tea, but they can also be used in capsules (use powdered herbs) or in a tincture or oil (use fresh herbs) to be rubbed into the temples and wrists. The instructions for making the tea follow. If you want to make an alcohol tincture or an oil, see the appropriate instructions in chapter 4: Medicine-Making Methods. Remember that when using fresh herbs, you need to triple the quantities.

Combine the roses, lemon balm, and violets together in a teapot. Pour 1 quart boiling water into the pot and allow the herbs to steep for 8 minutes. Add the motherwort to the teapot and brew 2 minutes more. Promptly strain the tea and check for sweetness using honey, stevia, or maple syrup. Drink it as often as you like.

Postpartum Tissue Care

Many husbands are prepared to help you breathe during labor, well advised on catching the baby, schooled on the importance of immediate breast-feeding, and ready to be loving and supportive fathers. The one thing they may not be expecting is the severity of the vaginal tear and the fact that your lower part is suddenly a wide-open, red injury. But this wound is very natural. The body copes with the passage of an enormous head quite gracefully; nevertheless, as a wound, it needs proper and consistent care. The perineum may tear; the labia and vaginal walls will stretch. In general, the lower pelvic region experiences a wonderful opening, a spreading, as if the force of the universe suddenly plunges into the material world (which, in fact, it does). It's a phenomenal and body-changing event for any woman, but make no mistake—it will heal. Whether or not you experience sutures or sewing, your lower region needs special care.

Herby Sitz Bath

A sitz bath is a special preparation of herbs to heal the perineum, labia, and vaginal tissues postpartum. These astringent herbs have the unique ability to "stitch" tissue back together and generate new skin. Many also fight bacteria, fungi, and other microbes that cause infection. They nourish, moisturize, and soothe, and this blend is a potent soak. The "tea" from these herbs can be poured into a bath, or—more convenient—placed in a special sitz bath tray available at pharmacies.

Combine the herbs and store them in the freezer bag. The night before you want to use them, place 1 cup dried herbs into a 1-quart glass jar. Cover them with boiling water to fill the jar and allow them to infuse overnight. In the morning, strain the liquid and store it in the refrigerator.

Measure equal parts of 3 or more of the following dried herbs to fill a 1-gallon freezer bag:

Calendula flowers

Comfrey leaves

Saint-John's-wort (leaves and flowers)

Red clover blossoms

Lady's mantle leaves

Sage leaves

Plantain leaves

Yarrow leaves

When ready to use, pour the liquid into a pan and gently heat it on the stovetop. When it's comfortably warm, pour it into the sitz bath tray on the toilet. Sit in the tray and soak for 10 minutes. Relax; envision your vaginal tissues as pink, healthy, happy tissues mending themselves, coming together seamlessly. Envision your uterus tightening up, and picture your cervix as a happy, healthy pink circle at the bottom of your uterus. Breathe deeply.

When you're finished, simply flush the tea down the toilet, and gently press an absorbent towel to your vagina to dry off. Repeat this bath several times daily for one to three weeks, or as needed. *Note:* This blend of dry herbs does not make a drinkable tea, because many of the herbs will dry up breast milk.

POSTPARTUM DEPRESSION AND MOTHER'S STRESS

Both new mothers and mothers with older children inevitably experience stress. Ecstatic visitors, helpful friends, a nervous husband, sleepless nights, and the questionable health of the mother and/or baby lead to anxiety and worry. Fatigue is common and is the body's way of encouraging you to sleep. By all means, sleep when your baby does. It's a precious time of growth and healing for you both.

Postpartum depression, on the other hand, is a severe, clinical form of anxiety that can overpower a woman's normal ability to cope. You may feel overwhelmed, sad, angry, bewildered, inferior, and exhausted; direct your frustration at other people and blame others; act irrationally; and in the most extreme cases, act violently toward yourself, your supporters, or even your baby or other children. This extreme depression requires immediate care from professional caregivers: physicians, psychologists, and other mainstream medical providers. It takes the full support of family and community to redirect your course back to the healthy path of motherhood so you can properly care for yourself and your family. You cannot do it alone; and your needs cannot be underestimated. Seek medical attention at once without fear or shame.

But not all depression is this severe—you may experience some discomfort, sadness, bleak feelings, or even question why you had this baby but still maintain control of your emotions and benefit from talking, crying, laughing. and sleeping. When depression is mild, it is useful to employ herbs. A number of herbs nourish the central nervous system in such a way that you will feel uplifted, gladdened, brightened. These are called the "Gladdening Herbs," and they include lemon balm, basil, lemon verbena, Saint-John's-wort, and borage, among others.

Motherwort Tincture

Motherwort tincture can be an effective and convenient remedy for a new mother dealing with mild depression. Motherwort is a wonderful herb; its name says it all: mother + wort (plant). This tincture can also address colic, because the bitter principles will be transferred through the breast milk. Motherwort is an effective remedy for the heart and is used for cardiac issues such as high blood pressure, weak or inconsistent heartbeat, and poor circulation (see chapter 12: Happy Heart for circulation-related recipes). Note: Don't consume this herb during pregnancy, as sometimes it acts as an emmenagogue, bringing on the menstrual cycle.

Yields ½ cup

½ cup fresh motherwort leaves, chopped
¼ cup 80 proof vodka
¼ cup water

Follow the instructions in chapter 4: Medicine-Making Methods for making an alcohol tincture, using a ½-pint glass jar in place of the 1-quart jar. Take ¼ teaspoon of this remedy 3 times daily, preferably in a small glass of Happy Sun Tea (the recipe follows).

MOTHERWORT
Leonurus cardiaca

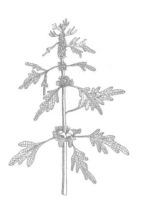

Long revered in European and Russian folk medicine, motherwort is renowned for two actions: (1) aiding congestion of the heart and strengthening heart tone, and (2) acting as a nervine tonic to soothe jangled nerves and even hysteria. Most herbalists today appreciate motherwort for its bitter principles, which are useful for digestive complaints (especially when prepared as a syrup). Many people find relief using motherwort for congestion in both the pelvic and the cardiac region, and I've used it countless times with blue vervain and lemon balm as a nonsedative nerve tonic.

Use caution when harvesting this prickly herb; it does not have thorns, but the flowers arise from sharp clusters that will puncture the skin. A member of the mint family, motherwort has the characteristic square stem and branching habit of peppermint, spearmint, apple mint, and catnip, but it tends to grow much taller. It spreads like wildfire and will send up dozens of new plants under the mother plant in only one season. It is the guardian plant of mothers (just as mugwort is the guardian of crones). Prepare it in small batches and brew for short lengths of time. Gather up your pluck and try it out.

Happy Sun Tea

Mild depression often responds to the therapeutic effect of flowers. A jar of sun tea steeping on the back porch looks beautiful and imparts the qualities of the herbs by way of a gentle, healing, and nourishing infusion. If you're using fresh herbs, triple the quantities.

Gather the herbs and combine them in a 2-quart glass jar. Cover them with enough fresh, cold water to fill the jar, and place the jar in a sunny spot. Allow it to steep all day, stirring occasionally. Strain the tea, and stir in honey to taste. Refrigerate it and drink it freely throughout the day.

Yields 2 quarts

4 tablespoons dried lemon balm leaves

4 tablespoons dried lemon verbena leaves and flowers

4 tablespoons dried borage leaves and flowers

4 tablespoons dried elder flowers

Honey

Elder Flower Hydrosol Spritzer

While writing this chapter, I kept hearing, "Use elder flower." I researched the use of elder flower for postpartum depression and did not find much in the literature. But the nagging was persistent, as if the Woman in the Elder wanted to be heard and would not be ignored. Perhaps she was used in ancient times and was a favorite among mothers and Wise Women, but her lore for postpartum depression has unfortunately been forgotten. Since elder flower and elderberry can be somewhat stimulating and can, in large doses, produce "evacuation" symptoms (they are often used to induce sweating during the flu), I decided to invite our dear elder flower into the repertoire for treating postpartum depression in an unobtrusive way: as a spray spritzer for the skin. Other flowers that work well for a postpartum spritzer are roses (any good-smelling variety), sweet orange blossoms, and violets.

Yields 1 pint

2 large handfuls fresh elder flowers

1 cup witch hazel

1 cup distilled water

1 teaspoon vegetable glycerin (optional)

In a pint jar, combine the flowers with the witch hazel and water. Cap tightly, label, and place on a sunny windowsill for 2 weeks. Strain, add the optional glycerin, and store in a small spray bottle. Spray it on your face, skin, and linens. *Note*: Vegetable glycerin can stain, so leave it out of the formula for use on linens.

BREAST MILK AND BREAST-FEEDING

Women's bodies are naturally built for making breast milk, that wonderfully nourishing liquid gold that sustains our babies and welcomes them into the world. Mother's first milk is colostrum, which is essential for Baby's first day of life. As he or she is born, the baby's body experiences a reduction in blood volume and its related die-off of red blood cells. These would toxify the baby's body if it weren't for colostrum's mild laxative effect, which helps the baby pass his or her first stool, called meconium. This laxative action also cleanses the baby's digestive tract. Colostrum is fantastically rich in nutrients: it contains proteins, vitamin A, and sodium chloride, in addition to being a storehouse of antibodies that will be the foundation of the baby's immune system. No artificial formula can match this.

Generally you can produce the colostrum and milk needed to feed your baby, but sometimes you may want to produce a greater quantity; for instance, if you are nursing twins or triplets, if you are a wet nurse, or if your body isn't supplying the quantity your baby needs. Often women who must take antibiotics prefer to increase their milk supply (and quality) in case the medication interferes with normal output. The greatest method for increasing milk supply is simply to nurse more frequently (and to drink plenty of fresh, clean water). The more you nurse, the more prostaglandin and milk your body produces. Occasionally, though, this isn't enough.

Thankfully, we have access to wonderful herbs called galactagogues, herbs that stimulate breast milk supply. These include Our Lady's milk thistle or blessed thistle (*Cnicus benedictus*), fennel, dill, and fenugreek.

The names themselves attest to the relief women throughout the ages have felt when their bodies finally start producing more milk thanks to these "blessed" plants.

HERBS THAT DRY UP BREAST MILK

Unless you are intentionally weaning your baby, as a breast-feeding mother, you will want to avoid consuming the following herbs. They are astringent and will dry up mucous and other bodily fluids, including breast milk: parsley, goldenseal, witch hazel, sage, yarrow, strawberry leaves, raspberry leaves, cranesbill root, lady's mantle, and calendula. Over-the-counter and prescription medications that dry up sinus congestion will also dry up breast milk.

Vineyard Herbs Breast Milk Fountain

This is a liquid tincture with concentrated extracts of herbs that boost your breast milk production. To remove the alcohol content when taking the tincture, simply drop the dose into a cup of hot tea and allow the alcohol to evaporate before drinking.

Fill a 1-pint jar with the herbs and cover completely with one-third vegetable glycerin, one-third vodka, and one-third apple cider vinegar. Follow the instructions in chapter 4: Medicine-Making Methods for making an alcohol tincture, and take it according to the dosage guidelines on pages 287–90.

Yields 1 cup

3 tablespoons dried or fresh blessed thistle

2 tablespoons fenugreek seeds

1 tablespoon fennel seeds

1 tablespoon nettle leaves

Vegetable glycerin

Vodka or brandy

Apple cider vinegar

Breast Milk Fountain Tea

Yields 1 quart

Combine any or all of the
following dried herbs to
make up ¾ cup:

Red clover blossoms

Nettle leaves

Raspberry leaves

Fenugreek seeds

Fennel seeds

Dill leaves

Alfalfa leaves

Hops flowers

This tea is the tastiest and best way to increase your milk supply. The herbs supply nourishment and satisfaction, in addition to flowing breast milk. Harvest as many of the following flowers and herbs as possible, and dry them on a newspaper or screen in a drafty, dim room. (Or purchase them ready-dried from a reliable source, such as a local health-food store or one of those listed in the Resources section at the end of this book.)

Combine the herbs in a 1-quart glass jar. Pour enough boiling water over them to fill the jar. Steep for 8 to 12 minutes. Strain the tea and pour into a thermos; drink it every time you nurse.

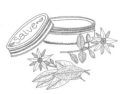

NIPPLE HEALTH

The following two recipes will soften sore and cracked nipples. Use fresh but lightly wilted herbs, and gently wash off the salve before nursing.

Nipple Nurse Salve 1

Yields 1 cup

½ cup fresh chicory leaves

½ cup fresh comfrey leaves

1 tablespoon fresh borage
flowers

1 cup lanolin, vegetable
oil, coconut oil, or shea
butter

This salve makes a deeply penetrating, healing balm for cracked skin tissues.

Place the herbs in a stainless steel or enamel pot on the stove. Spoon in the fat or oil, and gently warm it until it melts. Keep the heat low and stir frequently for 10 to 15 minutes. Strain the mixture, pour it into a small glass jar, and allow it to cool. The consistency will be semisolid, similar to room temperature coconut oil. Apply it as needed.

The herbs in this formula are soothing, moisturizing, and cooling for inflamed tissues.

Place the herbs in a stainless steel or enamel pot on the stove. Spoon in the oil and beeswax, and gently warm it until the wax melts. Keep the heat low and stir frequently for 10 to 15 minutes. Strain the salve and pour it into a bottle. Apply it as needed.

Yields 1 cup

½ cup dried marshmallow root

½ cup fresh red clover blossoms

¼ cup fresh rose petals or elder flowers

1 cup vegetable oil (such as sweet almond or jojoba)

¼ cup beeswax

WEANING AND DRYING BREAST MILK

Congratulations if you've been fortunate enough to breast-feed your baby! Perhaps you've spent months (or years) dutifully and happily supplying milk to your little one, day in and day out, and now you have a healthy, happy, chubby child to show for it. But you also might have a closet full of stained or stretched clothing, your nipples may be sagging or sore, and you may tend to smell like a Dairy Queen gone sour. Are you ready to stop nursing? To wean? To dry up the flow of milk? Or has your little one decided to wean on his or her own and now you're stuck with huge milk jugs on your chest? Ready to return to your size AA bra and get back to life as you once knew it?

Whatever method you use to wean your baby (I told my daughter my "nursies" didn't work anymore), you will need to dry your milk up safely and gracefully, since your body naturally wants to create more liquid gold. Take it slowly and don't expect your body suddenly to be milk-free. Often the weaning process takes weeks (both physically and emotionally), and this is best for both you and your baby. Milk jugs or no milk jugs, it's the relationship between you and your child that is most important.

These are natural ways to reduce or dry up the breast milk supply (be patient!):

- Reduce the number of times you breast-feed by once per day. This will gradually let your body (and baby) know that weaning has begun. Your body will begin to secrete prolactin-inhibiting factor (PIF) and will adjust accordingly.
- Reduce your intake of galactagogues, those wonderful herbs and foods that increase your milk supply. They include milk thistle, beer, and barley.
- Apply cabbage leaves. Gently pound the leaves to soften them, and apply them to your breasts either cold or warm, depending on your desire. They are soothing and wonderful for healing mastitis or nipple infections. (Some women who are allergic to sulfa-containing drugs such as Septra and Bactrim may react to cabbage.)
- The late herbalist Juliette de Bairacli Levy recommended using periwinkle (*Vinca major* and *V. minor*) internally, presumably as a tincture or tea, as well as externally as a poultice or compress made from the tea. It is a beautiful little trailing creeper with soft purple flowers, and you can use both the flowers and the leaves.

"No More Dairy Queen" Breast Milk Drying Formula

1 teaspoon dried yarrow

1 teaspoon dried sage

1 teaspoon dried parsley

This formula safely and naturally reduces your milk supply. It's safe to nurse while taking this preparation, but extra nursing will only prolong the weaning/drying process. It's best taken as a tea, but it can also be used as a tincture, as a compress, or in capsules. (For instructions on making an alcohol tincture, see chapter 4: Medicine-Making Methods.) Other herbs that will dry up milk include wild geranium (American cranesbill, or Geranium maculata) root and goldenseal. Goldenseal is on the United Plant Savers' At-Risk list, so don't use this valuable yet threatened herb unless absolutely necessary.

As a Tea

Combine the herbs in a jar. Cover 3 teaspoons herbs with 3 cups boiling water and steep 5 minutes. Strain. Add honey to taste; this brew is bitter and "dry" and will parch your mouth. For a less "parchy" brew, use only sage, and add mint or licorice if desired for taste. Drink hot, 1 cup 3 times daily.

As a Compress
Yields 3 cups

Follow the preceding instructions for making tea. Soak a clean cotton cloth in the tea and apply it warm or cold to your breasts for 10 minutes. If your baby is curious about what you're doing, let her help you hold the cloth in place. Tell her your breasts have done a good job nursing all this time and have given her wonderful milk. Now they're finished, and this tea and cloth is a nice way to say "thank you" to them.

As a Capsule

Combine equal parts dried powdered yarrow, sage, and parsley in a bowl. Spread them into gelatin capsules and take 3 to 7 daily. Combine this with the other therapies mentioned earlier.

GIFT IDEAS FOR MOTHERS-TO-BE

Many of the recipes and remedies in this chapter make wonderful gifts for new moms. Put together a gift basket with a container of Happy Sun Tea, a ceramic teapot, and a pottery mug. Make a tincture set with Motherwort Tincture and New Mother's Transition Tea. Or put together a gift basket with Herby Sitz Bath, Calendula-Beeswax Salve, and Elder Flower Hydrosol Spritzer. Include a soft baby's washcloth and a personal note with your basket, and you have a wonderful new-mother gift.

Chapter Six

———∘⟨⟩∘———

FOR INFANT AND CHILD

PARENTHOOD IS A WONDERFUL TIME of learning about new people: your baby, your spouse, and yourself. It can be a delightful experience, with hugging, kissing, singing, and cooing. Hopefully, there's adequate sleep too. Along with the wonderful joy of a new baby come discomforts that can often be remedied by using herbs. The following formulas are tried-and-true methods based on ancient tradition and personal experience. I have created and sold many of these remedies and have received positive feedback and thanks from relieved new mothers.

Remember that nursing infants absorb their nutrients through breast milk; when problems arise, consider your own diet and eliminate refined sugar, alcohol, and stimulants. Avoid possible allergens such as citrus fruits, cabbage, garlic, onion, soy, and wheat.

When making these preparations, create enough base formula to last several weeks; make your remedies for the day as you need them and store the final products in the refrigerator or a hot thermos. Though many of these remedies are specific to infants, a number of them are helpful for older children as well. When giving children medicine, you should generally reduce the adult dosage by two-thirds or follow the dosage guidelines on page 287–90.

CRADLE CAP

Medically known as seborrheic dermatitis, cradle cap is a nonharmful prob-lem commonly seen in infants. Most frequently observed on the scalp, cradle cap can appear in other oily or damp body locations, such as the face, neck, chest, and armpits. You may notice patchy scales or roundish, thick crusts on the scalp that are connected by a thin layer of skin tissue. Yellowish scales may attach to the hair shaft or dot the surface of the scalp, which may be reddish and inflamed. It may resemble dandruff or present as larger brown scales. Adults may experience this condition too, and the treatment (and cause) appear to be similar for both adults and children.

Traditionally accepted causes of dermatitis in children can include an overabundance of oil in the baby's or nursing mother's diet. If your baby has cradle cap, don't worry; simply follow the basic treatments given here and enjoy the one-on-one washing-and-combing time with your infant. Once his or her sebaceous glands are more fully developed, the problem will disappear.

Cradle Cap Oil

My son had cradle cap as an infant, and we managed to gradually remove the scales over the course of a few weeks. Basic treatments for infants include ap-plying an herbal oil to loosen the scales, then combing with an infant's comb to gently lift loose scales from the scalp.

Place the herbs in the oil, making sure the flowers are completely covered. Let the mixture steep for one month or more in a dark cabinet. Alternatively, gently simmer the mixture on low heat for 20 minutes. Strain the liquid, pour it into a clean bottle, and label it. Gently rub 1 teaspoon room-temperature oil (or more as needed) into the scalp in a circular motion and allow it to sit for an hour or overnight. Comb out loose scales and gently rinse the scalp, using the Baby Scalp Rinse that follows if the skin feels dry.

Yields 2 cups

1 cup fresh red clover
    blossoms
½ cup fresh mullein flowers
½ cup fresh plantain leaves,
    chopped
2 cups vegetable oil
    (such as apricot, sweet
    almond, canola, olive, or
    grapeseed)

Baby Scalp Rinse

Yields 2 cups

Combine any two of the
   following fresh herbs
   to equal 1 cup (or dried
   herbs to equal ¼ cup):
Elder flowers
Red clover blossoms
Plantain leaves
Violet flowers or leaves
Calendula flowers
2 cups water

This is a gentle wash for your baby's hair and scalp; the herbs are soothing, moisturizing, and mildly cleansing.

Place the herbs in a pot with the water and gently simmer over low heat for 10 minutes. Strain the liquid, pour it into a clean bottle, and label it. Allow it to cool. With your baby comfortably reclining in a baby bath, squirt or pour the rinse over his or her head. Gently pat the scalp dry with a towel and repeat as desired.

THRUSH/YEAST

Many excellent books detail the causes, symptoms, and remedies for yeast infections (*Candida albicans*), so we will not go into great detail here other than to say that babies who display thrush (white patches of yeast in the mouth) and women who experience yeast infections in the vagina or on the breasts are experiencing the effects of the same fungal infection. This can be passed from the baby's mouth to the nursing mother's nipples and back again, so it is essential to clean the nipples before and after each feeding. (For vaginal yeast infections, see also the Calendula Suppository in chapter 7: Especially for Women.)

Many people achieve good results by completing a liver cleanse or taking hepatic (liver-toning) herbs such as dandelion, yellow dock, and milk thistle. Pau d'arco is also a wonderful remedy for yeast infections, though you should not take it internally if you are pregnant or nursing; instead, make a water-based rinse (recipe follows) from the dried herb to apply topically or as a douche. Pau d'arco is too strong for your baby's mouth; for thrush, the Baby's Calendula Thrush Rinse (recipe follows) is best.

Candida Tincture for Nursing Mothers

This formula expels toxins and allergens from the liver that contribute to eczema and yeast infections. It is a safe and nourishing liver "cleanse" for nursing mothers (not for infants).

Follow the instructions in chapter 4: Medicine-Making Methods for making a vinegar tincture, using a 1-pint glass jar in place of the 1-quart jar. Cap the jar with a plastic lid and put it on a plate (sometimes vinegar tinctures ooze) in a dark cupboard for one month. Strain the liquid, pour it into a clean bottle, and label it. Use the dosage guidelines on pages 287–90.

Yields 1 cup

½ cup fresh dandelion root
¼ cup fresh yellow dock
    root
¼ cup fresh burdock root
¼ cup fresh nettle leaves
1 cup apple cider vinegar

Yeast Rinse

This rinse is formulated for use as a nipple rinse or a vaginal douche for the nursing mother who is dealing with a yeast infection or when the baby has thrush. The herbs are strong, traditional yeast-fighting herbs that, with consistent use, will clear up infections. As with all medicines, keep this mixture out of the reach of children.

In a teapot, submerge the herbs in the water and steep for 10 minutes. Strain the liquid through a cheesecloth and let it cool to body temperature. Dip a clean cotton cloth into the brew to apply topically or fill a douche bag for a vaginal remedy. This is an effective rinse when applied to the nipples, but your baby will find the taste bitter and disagreeable. Wash the nipples before nursing, then apply the rinse again afterward. For use with douche equipment, follow the manufacturer's instructions.

Yields 1½ cups

¼ cup dried pau d'arco
    herb
¼ cup dried calendula
    flowers
1 pint boiling water

Baby's Calendula Thrush Rinse

Yields 2 cups

1 cup fresh calendula petals

2 cups boiling water

Your baby's mouth is too sensitive for stronger yeast-fighting herbs, but calendula has earned its place as an effective yet safe herb for use with infants and children. Use fresh flower petals for best results.

In a teapot, submerge the herb in the water and steep for 10 minutes. Strain the liquid through a cheesecloth and let it cool to body temperature. Either gently wipe your baby's mouth with a cloth dipped in the liquid, or fill a rubber ball syringe and carefully squirt the liquid inside the baby's cheeks while he or she is in a reclined position and facing sideways or slightly downward. Support him or her securely and suck or wipe out any extra fluid.

EAR INFECTION/EARACHE

Almost all babies experience ear infections, since the ear canal is not fully developed yet, and its tight passageway can harbor bacteria, liquid, and even foreign objects. An otoscope is a valuable tool for determining how infected your baby's ear is and when it is appropriate to see the doctor. Not all ear infections require antibiotics—many respond well to herbal medicines. But some infections will persist; don't feel as though you've been defeated if you must administer antibiotics to your child.

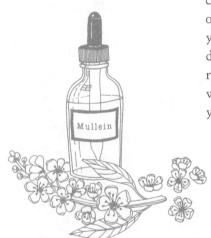

Mullein Flower Ear Oil

Mullein flowers earn their praise because they soothe, warm, and act on ear infections. I also like to add bacteria-fighting garlic, though the smell is strong. Store this oil in a small bottle in the refrigerator, heat a small amount for each use, and use the entire batch within a few days.

Coarsely chop the flowers, and place them—and the garlic, if using—in a pot. Pour the oil on top and gently simmer for 7 to 10 minutes. Be careful the oil doesn't burn, and stir the mixture frequently. Strain the liquid, pour it into a clean bottle, and let it cool to body temperature.

Carefully drop 2 to 5 drops into your baby's ear, massaging the ear and neck to guide the oil toward the inner tube. Let it sit for a moment, and then tip the baby's head onto a cloth to drain the ear canal. Repeat 3 to 6 times per day.

Yields ¼ cup

¼ cup (or a small handful) fresh mullein flowers

1 small clove garlic, freshly minced (optional)

¼ cup oil (olive, canola, or sweet almond)

WHEN TO USE COMMERCIAL MEDICINES

My philosophy of herbal medicine is that all healing methods have merit and value; they must be used correctly, with respect, and in the right circumstances. For instance, begin with healing foods, herbal infusions, teas, flower spritzes, flower essences, baths, long walks, and extra sleep. These are easy and barely intrusive, and children often respond well to them. If more intense methods are required, advance to other herbal therapies (tinctures, syrups, liniments, and so on) and external therapies (such as saunas and enemas). Finally, if these therapies haven't sufficiently treated the problem, you may feel perfectly justified in reaching for stronger (yet more invasive and consequently riskier) methods of healing that include surgery and antibiotics. The strength of following a natural therapy paradigm is that you allow your body to respond to milder forms of treatment first. This is essential.

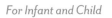

FEVERS AND COLDS

All children succumb to colds, fevers, and influenza eventually. These common occurrences stimulate a child's body to develop antibodies against further infection and strengthen the immune system for better health as an adult. But this doesn't make the infections any easier to deal with when your child is miserable, sick, sleepless, and cranky.

A fever is the body's response to a pathogen, an invader, or an illness. The body raises its core temperature in an attempt to "burn out" the invading germ, bacteria, or virus. Fevers are natural, though the body desperately wants to return to normal, and there are several natural ways to help your child's body do this.

Water Therapy

The body responds to changes in environmental temperature by adjusting its own temperature. Sometimes a quick change from hot to cold can trigger the necessary response in the body and reduce a fever. This therapy can be shocking (that's the point), and some children won't appreciate it; you know your child's temperament and can determine if water therapy is right for him or her.

Fill a bathtub with warm water, sprinkle in a handful of rose petals, and let your sick child sit in it. Let him play with the wet petals; they stick to the skin and can be fun. This might be enough for your child, but if you think a sudden temperature change will be of benefit, suggest that he get out of the bath and stand in a cool shower for 15 to 20 seconds. Make sure the water is not cold but just cool enough for a temperature difference to stimulate immune function. Return your child to the hot bath for 5 minutes, then wrap him in a warm towel or sheet and put him to bed.

Herbal Therapy

The following remedies are easy to make and will fill the house with a calming, comforting fragrance. Teas should be drunk as warm as possible, without burning your child's mouth or throat; give small doses frequently (every 20 to 30 minutes throughout the day, unless the child is asleep). See the dosage guidelines on pages 287–90 for specifics.

Elder Flower Tincture

Making an elder flower (Sambucus nigra, S. canadensis) tincture is easy and fragrant. Elder is prized as a safe fever reducer for children. Harvest the flowers by carefully snapping the large, soft flower head off the branch. At home, strip the little flower heads into a bowl; remove the large stem but don't worry about the tiny stems. Make this tincture in the early summer so you'll have a safe, effective autumn and winter fever remedy.

Stuff the flowers into the jar until it is full. Pour the glycerin, vodka, and water over the flowers, making sure they are completely submerged. Add extra vodka or water to bring the level to within ¼ inch of the rim. Cap the jar and shake it. Let the mixture steep for one month in a sunny windowsill and shake occasionally. Strain the liquid, pour it into a clean bottle, and label it. Follow the dosage guidelines on pages 287–90

Yields 1½ cups

Enough fresh elder flowers
   to completely stuff a
   1-pint glass jar
½ cup vegetable glycerin
½ cup vodka or brandy
½ cup distilled water

Children's Flu Syrup

Many of the Essential Herbs in this book are excellent cold and flu remedies, and they can be combined to make a delicious and effective syrup for children. Some are fever reducers; others are immune system strengtheners, adaptogens, or sedatives to support much-needed sleep. I recommend dried herbs for the following formula. If you're using fresh herbs, triple the amounts.

For this recipe, you'll need two separate pots, because you'll be making two separate concentrates. In one pot, combine the echinacea and elderberries; in the other, combine the catnip and elder flower. Cover each with 3 cups

Yields about 2½ cups

½ cup dried echinacea root
½ cup dried elderberries
½ cup dried catnip,
   chopped
½ cup dried elder flower
6 cups water
1 cup honey or maple syrup

water. Cover the pots with lids; place both on the stove. Simmer the echinacea/elderberries for 2 hours, stirring occasionally and skimming off the foam. After the first pot has been simmering for $1\frac{1}{2}$ hours, turn the heat on under the pot of catnip and elder flower. This allows the roots and berries in the first pot, which are harder, to cook longer; the more tender leaves and flowers in the second pot don't need as much time. When the pot of echinacea/elderberries has simmered the full 2 hours, remove both pots from the heat and strain the liquid into separate containers. This creates two strong infusions, and the liquid in each pot should be reduced to about 1 cup.

Combine the two teas and add the honey. Your syrup will be thin, tasty, and dark brownish or purple. Allow it to cool. Store the syrup in a glass bottle with a tight lid in the refrigerator. Follow the dosage guidelines on pages 287–90.

THE SIMPLER'S METHOD

Cold-and-flu syrups can be made with a great many ingredients, but I encourage you to use only a few herbs to get the job done. A young body responds well to simple remedies, and if your child displays an allergic reaction, you have a better sense of which herb to leave out next time. In the old days, this "purist" approach was that of the simpler, the apothecary who based remedies on one herb. It is a sensible and safe method for creating remedies for babies and children.

Children's Sleepytime Tonic

I created this formula years ago and frequently need to make new batches when it sells out. I've found that vegetable glycerin, which is overly sweet, sometimes counteracts the sedative effects of the herbs. For this reason, I advocate using half glycerin and half grain alcohol, such as vodka or brandy, or even abandoning the glycerin altogether in favor of the alcohol. If using alcohol is a concern, simply evaporate it by putting the tonic in a cup of hot tea (such as the Katama Chamomile Calming Blend). Make this remedy in advance and use it with other sleepytime tactics: soft music, dim lights, cuddling, and storytelling.

Yields approximately 1½ cups

¼ cup dried chamomile
¼ cup dried lavender
¼ cup dried catnip
⅔ cup vegetable glycerin
⅔ cup vodka
½ to 1 cup water

Follow the instructions in chapter 4: Medicine-Making Methods for making an alcohol tincture. Follow the dosage guidelines on page 287–90, and administer one dose an hour before bedtime and a second dose at bedtime.

Katama Chamomile Calming Blend Tea

This is a lovely, fragrant, satisfying sedative tea for children and adults. Over the years, I've experimented with the ingredients (sometimes using Saint-John's-wort, passionflower, or linden flower), and I've finally reached what I believe is a just-right formula. As the tea is naturally lightly sweet, additional sweeteners are rarely needed, but if your child insists, add a bit of honey to the cup. Note: Those with an allergy to ragweed species may experience an allergic reaction to chamomile.

Yields 1 quart

2 tablespoons dried chamomile
2 tablespoons dried spearmint
1 tablespoon dried catnip
1 teaspoon dried rose petals

Combine the herbs in a 1-quart glass jar. Pour enough boiling water over them to fill the jar. Let them steep for 5 to 8 minutes and strain the liquid, adding honey as desired.

Adults should drink this tea when it's hot, children when it's warm.

If you are breast-feeding a feverish and sleepless infant, it's best for you to drink the tea; the benefits will flow through the breast milk to relieve your child. (And you should sleep too!)

Eucalyptus-Menthol Respiratory Salve

Yields 1 cup

1 cup olive or canola oil

¼ cup beeswax

¼ teaspoon menthol crystals

10 to 15 drops eucalyptus essential oil

Like the famous vapor rub of old, you spread this salve directly on the chest so the invigorating, lung-healing vapors can be inhaled. It is a strong salve and may burn sensitive skin; test a little on the underside of the arm before using, and never use it on open wounds or broken skin. The ingredients can be found at most health food stores.

Follow the instructions in chapter 4: Medicine-Making Methods for making an herbal salve. Add the menthol crystals just as the beeswax melts. Then add the essential oil and immediately pour the mixture into a sealable glass container. Allow it to cool, then use as needed.

To use, spread the salve on the chest and then cover with a wet, warm washcloth. Allow your child to recline so her head is relaxed but above her chest and she can inhale the vapors. Let her rest this way for 10 minutes, then gently wipe off the salve with a wet cotton cloth. Repeat several times daily to ease nasal congestion, coughing, and a sore throat.

DIAPER RASH

Painful diaper rash can be caused by many factors: wet diapers; acidic foods in the mother's diet; allergies to soaps, detergents, or disposable diapers; excess humidity; and even the baby's stress. One of the best methods for treating diaper rash is to simply remove the diaper. That's right, get rid of them altogether, or at least for long periods of time, such as an entire afternoon. Let your baby's body be exposed to fresh air and sunlight. (If your child is old enough, this can assist in toilet training.)

Avoid hydrocortisone creams, as steroids can lead to future problems. Baby's immune system must be strengthened at this early age, not threatened or undermined. Zinc oxide has been used for decades and is effective, but gentler remedies, such as beeswax, are equally effective and completely natural. The following remedies use herbs to allay the irritating symptoms of diaper rash so both Baby and Mommy are more comfortable. (A health care practitioner must examine extremely stubborn diaper rash or open, puss-filled sores, as this could indicate a yeast infection or digestive disorder.)

Vitamin E Capsules

Sore skin with a rash often responds well to vitamin E. Purchase capsules and break one open; gently rub the oil on your baby's skin. Alternatively, break one capsule into a tablespoon of apricot kernel oil. Store it in a glass jar away from the baby's reach.

Evening Primrose–Vitamin E Oil

The lovely flower evening primrose opens only in the morning and evening; during the heat of the day, the blossom shuts tight. The oil extracted from the flower petals is high in gamma-linoleic acid (GLA), which has been lauded in clinical trials for healing a variety of ailments, including premenstrual syndrome, eczema, hyperactivity, and high blood pressure. This valuable oil makes a good addition to liquid vitamin E or a vegetable oil. Use it on diaper rash or any part of your baby's body that needs love, attention, massage, or moisture.

Yields ½ cup

1 cup packed fresh evening
   primrose flowers
½ cup vegetable oil
   (such as safflower,
   sunflower, grapeseed,
   or wheatgerm)

Press the flowers into a 1-pint glass jar. Pour the oil over the top and cap the jar; shake to ensure all the flowers are submerged in the oil. Let it steep for two weeks, shaking occasionally. Strain the liquid, pour it into a clean bottle, and label it. Gently rub it into the rash as needed.

Acidophilus

Some diaper rash can indicate a yeast infection. Lactobacillus acidophilus is a naturally occurring bacteria in the human digestive tract, and replenishing this bacteria (through the use of capsules, a liquid supplement, or some yogurts) can remedy yeast infections. Feed your baby ¼ teaspoon liquid acidophilus or 1 teaspoon plain unsweetened yogurt twice daily. If you are nursing, you should also consume an adult dose of acidophilus and should eat as much unsweetened yogurt as desired. If yeastlike symptoms continue, refer to the "Thrush/Yeast" section of this chapter or visit your health care practitioner.

Alkaline-Containing Foods

A diet high in acidic foods can alter the body's natural balance of intestinal bacteria to create an ultra-acidic digestive environment; this can sometimes result in diaper rash. Some baby foods are made with innocent-enough fruits, such as apples, but include added citric acid or ascorbic acid. If you're nursing, you should avoid acidic foods such as tomatoes, coffee, cranberries, olives, sauerkraut, tea, vinegar, and citrus fruits. Instead, include more alkaline-forming foods, such as molasses, kelp, fresh vegetables, avocados, corn, raisins, dates, and fresh coconut in your diet.

Calendula Beeswax Salve

Often considered one of the most effective and yet mildest of herbs, calendula (pot marigold) is an old remedy valued by our foremothers for treating their children's nicks, cuts, rashes, and boo-boos. The petals are easy to harvest and make a beautiful dark yellow or orange oil. By going a step further and turning this oil into a beeswax salve, you can create a nourishing, moisturizing, and effective water-barrier ointment to soothe your baby's diaper rash and protect fragile skin from further damage. Make a jar just for Baby's bottom and reserve another jar for rashes or wounds on other parts of the body so there is no risk of contamination or spreading germs.

Note: Red clover is an excellent substitute for calendula in this salve.

Follow the instructions in chapter 4: Medicine-Making Methods for making an herbal salve. You don't need to add scent, as this is one of the mildest salves you can provide for your baby.

Yields 1 cup

1 cup fresh calendula petals, picked from the flower head
1 cup vegetable oil (olive and canola are best)
¼ cup pure beeswax

Rose Body Powder

Excess moisture can cause diaper rash; soothing the skin and then drying the area are important. After making sure your baby's bottom is clean, gently towel-dry the area and sprinkle this soothing baby powder over the skin. Keep your baby's hands from touching it and spreading it to his eyes. This powder's base is arrowroot, a soothing herbal powder (unlike talc, which has been implicated in diseases).

Rose powder can be purchased from a high-quality herbal supplier (see the Resources section at the end of this book) or made in an herb or coffee grinder. To make your own, simply dry the rose petals in a shaded, well-ventilated part of the house; when they are crisp, spin them in the grinder. (Make sure it's a grinder you use only for herbs—it should be retired from its coffee grinding days!) Sift the pieces through a tight sieve and store them in a small jar with a tight lid. Rose powder stays fresh for one year when stored in a cool, dry place.

Yields approximately 1¼ cups

½ cup arrowroot powder
½ cup white kaolin powder
¼ cup powdered rose petals
1 to 3 drops rose essential oil (if desired)

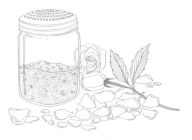

With a dry, long-handled spoon, gently combine the powders in a deep bowl. Add the essential oil if desired, and blend. Scoop the mixture into a powder container with a sifter lid (or a jar with a plain lid in which you poke holes using a small nail). Keep it in a dry place (not the bathroom!) and use as needed.

DIARRHEA

Children's digestive systems are young and developing. Imbalances happen, and most are ordinary and no cause for alarm. Diarrhea may indicate an intolerance of a certain food, or it may accompany a cold or influenza. By all means, if the symptoms persist for more than a few days, there is excessive blood in the stool, or your child spikes a fever, consult your health care practitioner. The best remedy is frequent breast-feeding for an infant or large amounts of water for a toddler. The following tea is astringent and will tighten loose tissues and retain water; this is useful because the biggest threat from diarrhea is dehydration.

Children's Raspberry Formula with Yarrow

Yields 3 to 4 cups

2 tablespoons dried raspberry leaves

1 tablespoon dried plantain leaves and/or root

1 tablespoon dried yarrow flowers and leaves

1 quart boiling water

Both raspberry leaves and yarrow leaves and flowers are astringent and have been used for centuries to address mild diarrhea. Plantain is soothing and, combined with raspberry and yarrow, creates a safe astringent formula for children of all ages.

Combine the herbs in a pot and add the water; steep for 10 to 12 minutes. Strain the liquid, pour into a clean bottle, and label it. This makes a rather astringent and bitter brew. Sweeten the formula as desired, and give it to your child by the teaspoonful every 15 minutes. (Nursing mothers: this is one tea you don't want to consume; the yarrow will dry up breast milk.) Store the bottle in the refrigerator and reheat it as needed.

It has a shelf life of 48 hours.

COLIC AND SLEEPLESSNESS/IRRITABILITY

Colic is an old-fashioned word for digestive upset. Children are considered colicky when they have upset tummies, are cranky, and can't sleep. Often gas is the culprit, and body massage can redirect trapped air. Foods can also cause colic, so it's wise to experiment to find out which foods your young one is not yet ready for. Babies often have trouble digesting garlic; onions; cabbage; fermented foods such as soy, tamari, sauerkraut; and acidic foods such as vinegar and citrus fruits (passed through the breast milk).

Lovely Catnip Tea

An easy, safe and effective remedy, catnip "tea" quickly relieves gas spasms, calms the tummy, and soothes the nerves, allowing a colicky baby to rest. For exhausted infants, this can be the make-it-or-break-it factor in finding a good night's sleep.

Yields 1 cup

2 teaspoons dried catnip
    leaves
1 cup boiling water

Place the herbs in a teapot and cover with the water; steep for 8 to 10 minutes. Strain the tea and add a touch of honey (only if baby is more than one year old). Let it cool slightly, then give the baby ¼ teaspoon at a time every 10 minutes. If you are breast-feeding, drink the tea frequently throughout the day and while nursing.

CATNIP
Nepeta cataria

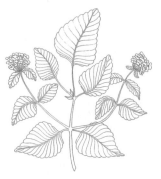

As a mint, catnip has the familiar square stem, branching habit, and white or pale purple flowers. It can quickly take over a garden, and like its cousins peppermint and spearmint, catnip (also called catmint) will form open, airy, bushlike herbal masses all over your growing beds. Both the stalks and the leaves are the color of silvery dust, and the flowers form clouds of tiny blossoms at the axil of each stalk.

Commonly called into action to entice and entertain kittens, catnip has the opposite effect on humans: it's calming and sedative. It makes a wonderfully effective bedtime tonic, and because it is safe, it is a favorite for children's remedies. Strip the leaves and flowers from the stalk and use it fresh, or pull up the plant and hang the entire herb from the rafters in an airy attic; a paper grocery bag hung around it and clamped at the top will catch drying leaves and seeds. When they are crisp, strip the leaves and store them in glass jars. The seeds germinate readily and can be sprinkled in the herb bed.

The following glycerite, which is simply a tincture made with glycerin instead of alcohol, can ease gas pains and help your baby's body excrete the digestive enzymes necessary for metabolizing new foods. You can also use these herbs to make a strong tea for yourself or to be dropped right on Baby's tongue.

Yields 1½ cups

¼ cup fresh ginger, chopped

¼ cup fresh lemon balm leaves

¼ cup fresh chamomile flowers

¼ cup fresh plantain leaves

1 cup water

½ cup vegetable glycerin

2 tablespoons brandy

Combine the herbs in a 1-pint glass jar. Add the water, vegetable glycerin, and brandy, filling the jar to the top, using extra glycerin if needed. Cap the jar tightly, and steep for two weeks. Strain the liquid, pour it into a clean bottle, and label it. You can use it in several ways: drop it right on Baby's tongue; hold the dropper beside your nipple while nursing and gently squeeze the bulb; drop it into the baby bottle; or take an adult dose yourself to pass it through your breast milk. Consult the dosage guidelines on pages 287–90 for specifics.

A beautiful wildflower and valuable medicinal herb, the violet (Viola odorata) is among nature's loveliest gifts. Violet leaves and flowers have been used in our herbal heritage for healing headaches, hot nervous conditions, external wounds, internal swelling, breast tenderness, and respiratory congestion. Collect the flowers to make this honey or a sun tea. For more ideas on using violets, see Susun Weed's charming book Healing Wise. *You shouldn't give honey to infants until they are one year old, as their immune systems cannot yet fight off any botulism spores that may be in it.*

Yields 1 cup

3 cups packed fresh violet flowers

1 cup honey

In a stainless steel or glass pot, gently heat the honey until it melts. Add the flowers and steep on low heat for 10 minutes. Strain the honey into a jar, cap it tightly, and label it. Give a few drops to your child every 30 minutes or so, or drizzle it onto his finger and allow him to suck it. You can also stir this honey into a cup of Katama Chamomile Calming Blend Tea (see the "Fevers and Colds" section of this chapter) for sweetness. Stored in the pantry, this honey will keep up to one year.

Baby Massage Oil

Yields 1½ cups

Combine any of the
following fresh but
lightly wilted flowers to
make 1 cup:

Calendula petals

Elder flowers

Evening primrose flowers

Lavender flowers

Red clover flowers

Rose petals

Violet flowers

1 to 1½ cups vegetable oil
(something luxurious
but mild, such as sweet
almond oil or apricot
kernel oil)

Vitamin E capsule
(optional)

Massage can be a wonderful experience for both you and your baby. Gently rub her arms, legs, hands, and feet; when massaging her belly, rub in a clockwise motion starting at the lower right side of her abdomen (your lower left) and going up, across, and down. This follows the direction of the large intestine, small intestine, and colon, and the motion can ease digestion. These herbs make a delightful, nourishing baby massage oil.

Follow the instructions in chapter 4: Medicine-Making Methods for making an herbal oil, using a 1-pint glass jar in place of the 1-quart jar. After straining the herbs from the oil, break open the vitamin E capsule and add its contents to the oil, if desired.

Before using, warm the oil in your hands. This is a great time for cooing and singing. Even better, while you're massaging your baby, have your spouse massage you!

Children's Nighttime Tummy Tincture

This is a mellow and calming formula that eases tension, upset tummies, stress, and chronic fear. To evaporate the alcohol, simply place the dose in a cup of warm (preferably catnip) tea.

Follow the instructions in chapter 4: Medicine-Making Methods for making an alcohol tincture, using a 1-pint glass jar in place of the 1-quart jar. Use the dosage guidelines on pages 287–90. It is best given half an hour before bedtime.

Yields 1 cup

¼ cup fresh chamomile
¼ cup fresh catnip
¼ cup fresh rose petals
¼ cup fresh wild lettuce
   (optional)
½ cup grain alcohol (such
   as vodka or brandy)
½ cup water

Lemon Balm Infusion

This is a heavenly, fragrant herbal tea that's perfect for little ones to sip.

Place the herb in a 1-quart glass jar and pour enough boiling water over it to fill the jar. Steep for 8 to 10 minutes, then strain. Sweeten the tea with honey or maple syrup to taste, and allow it to cool enough for your child to sip. If he balks, letting him use a straw sometimes does the trick.

Yields 1 quart

4 to 6 tablespoons dried
   lemon balm
Honey or maple syrup

Calming Baby Bath

Soothing and fragrant, this combination of herbs is a welcome and calming addition to your child's bath routine. Pour this infusion directly into the bathwater before your child gets in.

Yields approximately 2 quarts

¼ cup dried lavender flowers
¼ cup dried rose petals
2 tablespoons dried catnip

Combine the herbs in a 2-quart glass jar and pour enough boiling water over them to fill the jar. Cover it tightly and steep for 8 to 10 minutes. Strain the infusion, allow it to cool slightly, and add the entire infusion to the bath.

Lavender-Catnip Bedtime Buddy

½ cup dried lavender
½ cup dried catnip
2 6-inch squares of soft cloth such as cotton, flannel, or velvet
Markers (optional)

If you're sew-inclined, stitching a small buddy for your little one to cuddle is a great way to bring confidence to that scary thing we call bedtime. Fill the buddy with fragrant lavender and dried catnip; this will lull your child to sleep.

Make your buddy any shape you wish; simple people shapes about the size of your hand are fun and require no pattern, just an attempt at symmetry. Draw your shape on the wrong side of two pieces of fabric and cut it out. Draw eyes or a face on the right side of your fabric if desired. Lay the fabric pieces together, right sides facing, and stitch all the way around ⅝ inch from the edge; leave about 2 inches unstitched. Turn the buddy right-side out and fill it with herbs, pushing them into whatever appendages you've created. Stitch the remaining opening closed.

TEETHING

Often Baby's first experience with pain and discomfort, teething is a natural occurrence we all live through. There are several natural remedies to ease little ones' first experience with growth and maturity.

Katama Chamomile Calming Blend Tea

Listed earlier in the "Fevers and Colds" section, this tea is also a wonderful aid for babies dealing with teething. Follow the previous instructions for brewing and give your baby a teaspoonful every 15 minutes. If possible, rub a little of the tea on her gums. If she doesn't want you to mess with her mouth, try dipping her gummy toy (or anything she sucks on) in the tea. This is also a good tea for Mom and Dad to drink to relieve the stress of dealing with a cranky child!

Numbing Teething Oil

Most of the teething oils found in stores and pharmacies are far too strong for a baby. They contain clove oil or cinnamon oil, which are both analgesic (pain relieving) but intense. These strong oils are better when diluted—a drop of clove oil can be plenty for a teething baby—and they are best mixed with other oils to improve their flavor.

Mix all of the ingredients together in a small glass or ceramic bowl, whisking until blended. Store the oil in a small jar in the refrigerator for up to 3 weeks. Gently rub it on your baby's gums as needed.

Yields 1 tablespoon

2 drops rose essential oil or hydrosol (flower water)
2 drops mint essential oil or hydrosol (flower water)
1 drop clove essential oil
1 tablespoon mild vegetable oil (such as safflower or sunflower)

Rose Spritzer

Yields ⅓ cup

⅓ cup distilled water
5 to 15 drops rose
   essential oil

Roses are flowers of the gods. Their heavenly scent is calming and soothing for a little child with teething pain. This spritzer, or spray, is easy to make and can be sprayed directly on your baby's face or body (avoiding the eyes), or misted on clothing, linens, or pillowcases. Older children can practice their dexterity by learning to push the button or trigger on the spray bottle. Make sure they don't spray it in their eyes (or those of the cat or dog) and let them spritz away.

Combine the liquids in a bottle with a spray top. Store it in the fridge for a cool spray on hot days and to prolong its potency. It has a shelf life of approximately one month when refrigerated. *Note:* ¼ teaspoon vegetable glycerin can be added for skin-soothing properties, but the glycerin may stain clothing and linens.

Chapter Seven

ESPECIALLY FOR WOMEN

Women put so much into life: raising families, caring for elders, organizing schools, participating in politics, and running businesses. Of course, men do all of this as well, but women have special organs and systems that suffer the brunt of heavy hormonal changes and childbearing that remind us to take extra care of our bodies.

The recipes in this chapter address common problems women experience in the general course of life, many of which can be corrected with proper diet; adequate sleep; good nutrition; and herbs that affect the hormonal, nervous, and digestive systems. Give your body time to adjust to these herbal remedies, as most herbs require consistent use over time to bring about the fullest positive change.

ANEMIA

Women bleed from menarche, which is the first menstrual period for a young woman, all the way through menopause, which is the cessation of the menstrual cycle. We sometimes bleed a lot, and as a result, we can lose valuable iron. This can result in lethargy, weakness or inactivity, a loss of purpose, and easy bruising. Thankfully, some herbs are rich in easily assimilated iron that can replenish our supplies and keep us vibrant, strong, and free of bruises.

IRON-RICH FOODS

The most easily accessible iron is found in animal flesh (heme iron); vegetable sources supply non-heme iron that requires bitters to absorb properly. Many herbalists recommend taking iron (via herbs or supplements) with the bitter herb gentian. Ingesting fresh oranges and other citrus fruits, orange juice, and straw-berries can also help the body use non-heme iron from iron-rich sources; the best of these sources include: amaranth, dried apricots, bladderwrack, chlorella, dandelion leaf and root, dates, kelp, lamb's quarters, licorice, pumpkin seeds, blackstrap molasses, mustard greens, nettle, oatstraw and bran, parsley, prunes, raisins, sarsaparilla, thyme, watercress, and yellow dock.

Anemic women should avoid alcohol and caffeine (which sap iron from the body). Also, foods that inhibit iron absorption, such as soy, should be eaten sepa-rately from high-iron foods. Cooked spinach contains 3.5 milligrams of iron per cup, but it also contains oxalic acid (as does our tangy wood sorrel herb). Oxalic acid can reduce iron absorption in the body, so it's best to enjoy cooked spinach with iron absorption enhancers, such as bitters, foods rich in vitamin C, and foods containing deadly nightshade such as tomatoes and potatoes.

Iron-rich foods and herbs are much healthier choices than store-bought, labo-ratory-created iron supplements that often cause constipation. Dandelion greens contain as much iron as spinach and twice as much as collard greens. A delicious 3½-ounce serving of raw dandelion greens contains 17 percent of the U.S. recom-mended daily allowance for iron.

Moon Time Vinegar Tincture

The purpose of this formula is to increase the iron supply in the blood to prevent or reverse anemia. It's a good opportunity to use fresh herbs and roots; use the best-quality vinegar you can find.

Combine the chopped, cleaned herbs and roots, and place them in a 1-quart glass jar. In a pan, gently heat the vinegar; when it reaches a simmer, pour it over the herbs in the jar. Cover the mixture with enough fresh water to bring the liquid to within ¼ inch of the rim. Cap the jar and label it. Steep for two weeks or longer. Strain the liquid, and press the herbs firmly to get out as much valuable liquid as possible. Compost the leftover herbs. Add the molasses to the liquid, and pour it into a clean, labeled bottle. Use the dosage guidelines on pages 287–90.

Yields 2 cups

½ cup fresh dandelion
  root, chopped (about 1
  small root)
½ cup fresh dandelion leaves
½ cup fresh yellow dock
  root, chopped
½ cup fresh nettle leaves
  (or ¼ cup dried)
½ cup fresh parsley leaves
  (or ¼ cup dried)
2 cups apple cider vinegar
2 tablespoons blackstrap
  molasses

Iron-Rich Salad Dressing

This is an easy-to-use, delicious salad dressing that's wonderful on green leafy salads and steamed vegetables. It's a nice way to add extra iron to your diet. Make the prepared vinegar base first and combine it with oil when making your salad.

Gently heat the vinegar in a pot and simmer for 7 to 8 minutes. Chop the herbs finely with a knife and place them in a 1-quart glass jar with a plastic lid. Pour the hot vinegar over the herbs, and place the jar in a cool, dark cabinet on top of a plate. Steep for two weeks, shaking occasionally. Strain the liquid, pour it into a clean bottle, and label it. This is your prepared vinegar base.

Yields about 2 cups

2 cups apple cider vinegar
1 cup fresh dandelion
  leaves, chopped
3 tablespoons fresh
  parsley, chopped
3 tablespoons fresh
  watercress, chopped
3 tablespoons fresh nettle
  leaves, chopped

To make the dressing, combine ½ cup prepared vinegar with 1½ cups good-quality olive (or safflower, sunflower, or canola) oil. Add salt and pepper to taste, mix well, and serve. Reserve the rest of the vinegar in the refrigerator and use as needed.

It has a shelf life of approximately six months when refrigerated.

❧ Delicious Mineral Decoction

Yields 2 cups

3 tablespoons fresh
   dandelion root,
   chopped (or
   1 tablespoon dried)
3 tablespoons fresh
   wild sarsaparilla root,
   chopped (or 1 table-
   spoon dried)
3 tablespoons fresh yellow
   dock root, chopped (or
   1 tablespoon dried)
2 cups water
Molasses or maple syrup,
   to taste

Rich in healthy minerals such as calcium, magnesium, and iron, this strong-tasting beverage is a hearty nourisher when the body feels weak or depleted.

Follow the instructions in chapter 4: Medicine-Making Methods for making an herbal decoction. Store in a lidded glass jar in the refrigerator and drink ½ cup 3 times daily, during menstruation or anytime extra iron is needed.

BONE HEALTH

Strong bones are a result of lucky genetics and a good diet, not to mention a healthy, active lifestyle that includes appropriate weight-bearing exercise. The body is continually breaking down bone mass and replenishing it with fresh bone material; some estimates show that 20 percent or more of an adult's bone mass is replaced every year. Cigarette smoking affects the body's absorption of critical minerals such as calcium and silica that are necessary to build and maintain a strong skeleton. Herbs high in calcium and silica include nettle, red clover, alfalfa, horsetail, oatstraw, and raspberry. To promote calcium absorption, take vitamin D supplements at the same time. (See also the "Calcium" section in chapter 5: For the Expectant and New Mother.)

It's no wonder this strong, rich tea tastes so good; it's full of delicious herbs that are naturally sweet and pleasant. But it is also surprisingly nutritious— a drinkable, natural mineral supplement that is high in calcium, potassium, iron, magnesium, and zinc. Use dried herbs for this recipe.

Combine all the herbs in a 2-quart glass jar. Pour enough boiling water over them to cover them. Cover the jar and steep overnight. Strain the tea into a thermos, sweeten to taste, and drink it freely. Refrigerated, this tea will keep 2 to 3 days.

Yields 1 quart

2 tablespoons dried nettle leaves
2 tablespoons dried oatstraw
2 tablespoons dried red clover
2 tablespoons dried dandelion leaves
2 teaspoons dried alfalfa
2 teaspoons dried chamomile
2 teaspoons dried raspberry leaves
2 teaspoons dried violet leaves

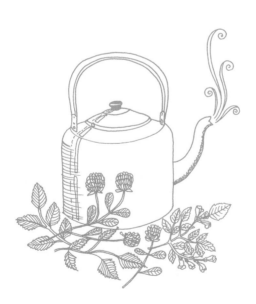

Herbal Nut and Seed Butter

Yields 2 cups

Choose one or combine
several of the following
shelled, raw nuts and
seeds to make 2 cups:

Hazelnuts

Pecans

Walnuts

Chia seeds

Sesame seeds

Almonds

Very high in protein and strengthening minerals, these nuts and seeds make wonderful "butters." George Washington Carver first introduced peanut butter after he roasted and ground raw peanuts; today, we are fortunate to have easy access to a variety of the world's nuts and seeds and can easily create homemade nut butters of our own. Roasting brings out the rich flavor of the nuts or seeds, and grinding them into butter makes them easy to enjoy with snacks or meals.

Spread the seeds or nuts on a cookie sheet and roast them in a preheated oven set at 350º F for 10 minutes, until they are fragrant and darker. With a hand grinder or a food processor, grind into a thick butter or paste. If the mixture is dry, add a small amount of sunflower oil. Serve the butter on crackers or whole wheat bread with honey or jam for a calcium-rich treat.

Refrigerated, it has a shelf life of approximately one month.

Savory Calcium Sprinkle

Yields approximately 1½ cups

3 tablespoons celery seeds

3 tablespoons dill seeds

3 tablespoons dried nettle
leaves

3 tablespoons dried
oregano

2 tablespoons dried fennel
seeds

2 tablespoons dried savory

Sprinkle this calcium-rich blend over garlic toast, soup, or bruschetta for a savory flavor.

Combine the herbs and store them in a glass jar with a tight-fitting lid, in a tin, or in an herb jar with a sifter top.

This blend has a shelf life of four months.

This blend of herbs is delicious over oatmeal, in granola, and in breads. Sprinkle it on many dishes for an uplifting, fragrant, and calcium-rich addition.

Combine all the ingredients and store them in a glass jar with a tight-fitting lid, in a tin, or in an herb jar with a sifter top.

    This blend has a shelf life of approximately six months.

Yields approximately ¼ cup

3 tablespoons poppy seeds

¼ teaspoon powdered cinnamon

¼ teaspoon powdered nutmeg

BREAST HEALTH

Breasts are a complex system of lymph glands and fibrous tissues that, when functioning properly, help the immune system relieve and discharge fluids. When inflamed, however, these glands can become painfully swollen, and the tissues can harbor dangerous cancerous growths. To keep breast tissues and lymph glands healthy, follow a healthy diet, drink fresh water, and practice monthly breast exams so that any new growths or lumps can be assessed. Discuss any new, hard, or painful lumps with your health care practitioner.

Nipple Moisturizing Oil

Yields 1½ cups

2 tablespoons dried
marshmallow root

2 tablespoons fresh red
clover

1 tablespoon fresh rose
petals or elder flowers

1 tablespoon fresh chicory
leaves

1½ cups vegetable oil (such
as sweet almond or
jojoba)

*This thick oil softens sore skin and is helpful for new mamas or any woman
with dry, cracked nipples.*

Follow the instructions in chapter 4: Medicine-Making Methods for making an herbal oil. Apply the oil with your fingers or a cotton ball daily
to soothe the skin, make your nipples and breasts supple and elastic, and
encourage proper blood flow.

Store the oil in a cool cupboard. It has a shelf life of approximately two
months.

Cyst-Dissolving Oil

Yields 1¼ cups

2 tablespoons fresh
plantain leaves,
chopped

2 tablespoons fresh red
clover blossoms

1 tablespoon fresh mullein
leaves, chopped

1¼ cups vegetable oil (such
as sweet almond or
jojoba)

*Many herbalists use herbs topically to dissolve cysts and loosen fibrous tissues
directly beneath the surface of the skin. Poke root is a great herb for this, as it
has the reputation for pulling materials up through the flesh and out through
the skin. However, since this can be a scary and painful process, I've elected to
include a recipe made with the Essential Herbs that are traditionally known
for dissolving growths and encouraging blood flow beneath the skin surface.*

Follow the instructions in chapter 4: Medicine-Making Methods for making an herbal oil. Apply the preparation to the entire breast with your
fingers in a circular motion. Take this opportunity to lie back; relax; and
visualize the cyst dissolving under the skin, being absorbed by the body,
and turning into healthy, vibrant tissue.

LYMPH SYSTEM

The complex lymph system traverses the entire body. Lymph tissues and lymphoid follicles are associated with the immune and digestive systems and can be found in the spleen, tonsils, thymus, bone marrow, and other organs. Interestingly, lymph fluid travels through the lymphatic vessels in a one-way direction toward the heart. This amazing vessel network can trap cancerous cells and destroy them, but sometimes cells are not destroyed and the cancer can travel through the lymph network to other nodes that can harbor secondary tumors. Herbalism can help keep the lymph fluids flowing freely. Herbs such as cleavers (*Gallium aparine*) or ladies' bedstraw (*Galium verum*) have historically been prized for "decongesting" the lymph system and allowing the fluids to travel.

Love Your Lymph System Tea

This formula uses alterative herbs (herbs that can alter the body's response to stress) such as red clover, as well as diuretic herbs such as cleavers. This combination tones and drains the lymph system, fights abnormal cell growth, and encourages blood flow. Use this tea for tonsillitis, cysts, ulcers, and tumors.

Combine the herbs in a 1-quart glass jar. Pour enough boiling water over them to cover them. Steep for 15 to 30 minutes, tightly covered. Strain the tea well, sweeten with honey to taste, and drink 2 to 4 cups daily for up to two weeks. Refrigerate leftover tea and use within 24 hours.

Yields 1 quart

4 tablespoons dried
   cleavers
2 tablespoons dried red
   clover
1 tablespoon fresh ginger
   (or ½ teaspoon
   powdered)
½ teaspoon dried
   calendula
Honey

Wild Herbflower Tea

Yields 1 quart

2 tablespoons dried red
    clover blossoms
1 tablespoon dried gotu
    kola leaves
1 tablespoon dried
    lemongrass or lemon
    balm
1 tablespoon dried
    spearmint or
    peppermint
Honey

This is a lovely, fragrant brew—nourishing and full of vitamins and minerals. I love to harvest fresh red clover blossoms and dry them on a screen, then blend them with herbs that add a little punch, like lemongrass or lemon balm. Because both the gotu kola and lemon balm are traditionally used to improve memory and focus, this is a wonderful tea to drink during exams or work on important projects.

Combine the herbs in a 1-quart glass jar. Pour enough boiling water over them to fill the jar. Steep for 12 to 15 minutes. Strain the tea and sweeten it with honey to taste, though this tea is naturally sweet. Enjoy 2 to 3 cups daily, refrigerating any leftover tea for up to 24 hours.

FERTILITY

The many reasons why we sometimes can't reproduce are too numerous to cover in this book: genetics, hormonal inconsistencies, poor health, pollutants, environmental toxins, stress . . . A qualified health care practitioner can diagnose problems and pinpoint strategies to help you successfully conceive a child. (And if not, adopting a baby, toddler, or older child is a highly rewarding way to contribute to family—both yours and the global kind.)

If you want to conceive but it's not happening, rejoice in the fact that you get to have sex as often as you wish, and follow these guidelines:

- Eat a diet that is not only adequate but also nourishing. Think fertile: green, juicy, and fresh. Eat foods bursting from the vine and fresh from the field and garden, foods that mirror the rainbow and include every color. Include juicy, squeezable fruits and vegetables; seaweeds; herbs; lean meats; round grains; and plenty of fresh water in your daily intake.

· Completely avoid smoking, drinking alcohol and caffeine, and working in a polluted environment. Does your office smell of ink toner cartridges? Does the florist where you work use chemical stabilizers for the flowers? Make your body a temple of fertility by steering away from unhealthy substances.

· This doesn't mean make your body a temple of purity. Purity is different. You needn't be smooth, pure, and innocent in order to conceive. Quite the contrary: a wild, active, and adventurous woman can be quite fertile—Mother Earth is a prime example.

· Consider how active you are. Overactivity is just as unproductive as underactivity. Work with your health care practitioner (and supportive family) to determine an exercise and athletic schedule that is right for you.

· Think positively. Be proactive, imaginative, creative, happy, grateful, and joyful. Spread kindness far and wide. A happy heart makes for a fertile womb. (In other words, reduce your stress, worry, and anxiety, which can produce hormones that limit conception.)

· Indulge in nourishing, mineral-rich, hormone-balancing herbs. These can be delicious teas, supplements, capsules, or tinctures that sustain your body and balance your reproductive system. Instead of looking at it as "taking your medicine" or following a regimen, consider it a treat for the temple of your body: delicious teas are gifts for both you and your upcoming baby.

Fertili-Tea

Yields 1 quart

2 tablespoons dried red clover

1 tablespoon dried chaste tree berries

1 tablespoon dried lemon balm

1 tablespoon dried nettle leaves

Red clover is a prime alterative herb used to bring the body into balance and alter the way it reacts to stress. It's also rich in minerals and contains phytoestrogens that can balance hormones. Chaste tree berries (Vitex agnus-castus) stimulate the pituitary gland to increase or decrease estrogen and (especially) progesterone as needed. Many herbalists use chaste tree berry to help patients "balance" the body's hormones after using birth control pills. Lemon balm is a wonderful nervine.

Combine the herbs in a 1-quart glass jar. Pour enough boiling water over them to fill the jar. Steep overnight. Strain the tea in the morning and drink it freely, refrigerating any leftover tea for up to 24 hours.

Nourishing Mama Tonic

This combination of herbs is at once calming and nutritious, and it will act as a gentle digestive tonic as well. Note: The tea is bitter.

Yields approximately 1 cup

2 teaspoons dried alfalfa leaves

2 teaspoons dried nettle leaves

1 teaspoon motherwort

½ cup vodka or brandy

½ cup water

As a Tincture

Follow the instructions in chapter 4: Medicine-Making Methods for making an alcohol tincture. Drop the correct dose into a cup of warm tea and allow time for the alcohol to evaporate before drinking.

As a Tea

Follow the instructions in chapter 4: Medicine-Making Methods for making an herbal infusion with the nettle and the alfalfa. Add the motherwort in the last few minutes of steeping to avoid excessive bitterness. Strain the tea, sweeten to taste, and drink it freely. Refrigerate any leftover tea for up to 24 hours.

HERPES

For remedies related to herpes and cold sores, see chapter 11: Healing Wounds.

HORMONES AND PREMENSTRUAL SYNDROME

Women's hormones fluctuate—that's what they do. They naturally cycle with the moon so that sometimes we feel "up" and sometimes "down." Women are especially vulnerable to low feelings during the luteal phase after ovulation when estrogen has plummeted and progesterone is spiking. Some women experience painfully swollen breasts, grumpiness, mood swings, an inability to think clearly, cramps, a "downward-drawing" feeling, and other irritating symptoms. Others experience dangerous feelings such as extreme depression and suicidal tendencies. Such symptoms, of course, require the intervention of qualified caregivers and a supportive community, but herbs can be useful and surprisingly effective for the milder symptoms.

Premenstrual syndrome (PMS) is a complex set of issues involving hormonal fluctuations in the menstrual cycle. Women experience the symptoms differently, but emotions are generally volatile, raw, and wildly fluctuating. Many women experience emotional roller-coasters that involve crying—for no particular reason, because they're happy, because something slightly sad happens, or because they just can't get through the next

Yields 1 quart

3 tablespoons dried nettle leaves

3 tablespoons dried alfalfa leaves

1 tablespoon motherwort

Sweetener, such as honey, stevia, or maple syrup

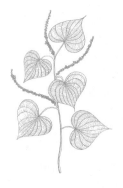

sentence without breaking down in tears. They insist that their husbands and boyfriends leave them alone, then cry because the men have left.

A diet high in the mineral magnesium can help reduce these symptoms. Foods such as lima beans, soybeans, garbanzo beans (chickpeas), spinach, yogurt, pumpkin seeds, bran muffins, and buckwheat pancakes contain high levels of easily digestible magnesium. In addition, sufferers can take a strong multivitamin and mineral supplement with 320 milligrams magnesium daily throughout the month to balance hormonal swings.

Wild Yam PMS Jam

Yields 3 to 4 cups

¼ cup dried wild yam root, chopped

¼ cup dried black cohosh root, chopped

2 tablespoons dried motherwort

2 tablespoons dried crampbark

2 tablespoons dried chaste tree berries

1 tablespoon dried dandelion leaves

3 cups grain alcohol (such as vodka or brandy)

1 cup distilled water

I've had husbands ask me if I will sell their wives this tincture by the gallon. Women respond well to this combination of nervine, tonic, and hormone-balancing herbs. It's a combination of my Essential Herbs with a few slightly more exotic herbs you can purchase at a health food store.

Follow the instructions in chapter 4: Medicine-Making Methods for making an alcohol tincture. Once strained, it will last for several years and yield a consistent supply for your monthly needs.

Begin taking doses (see the dosage guidelines on page 287–90) approximately 5 to 6 days before you expect PMS symptoms to begin, and continue taking until menstruation has ceased. Resume this pattern for each cycle.

Similar in effect to the Wild Yam PMS Jam, this tasty brew will satisfy and calm you throughout your premenstrual time.

Lightly crush the chaste tree berries in a mortar and pestle or a food processor. Combine the berries with the herbs and place them in a 1-quart glass jar. Pour enough boiling water over them to fill the jar. Steep for 12 to 15 minutes. Strain, store in a thermos or jar, and refrigerate any leftover tea for up to 24 hours.

Drink 1 to 3 cups daily, beginning several days before your PMS symptoms are expected and continuing through the first full day of menstruation (or later). Resume this pattern for each cycle.

Yields 1 quart

2 tablespoons dried chaste
  tree berries
2 tablespoons dried
  dandelion leaves
2 teaspoons dried red
  clover blossoms
1 teaspoon dried nettle
  leaves
1 teaspoon dried holy basil
  (*Ocimum tenuiflorum*,
  or tulsi)

MENOPAUSE

Unlike cyclical hormone changes, menopause is the permanent cessation of all menstrual cycles. But menstruation doesn't just end all at once; it ceases gradually as the pituitary and other glands no longer stimulate hormones in a predictable pattern. Follicle-stimulating hormone is no longer needed since the egg is no longer needed, but the body takes its time in ending this process. Some women experience symptoms over the course of a year; for others, it can last several years.

Many women experience no symptoms at all and enjoy their "crone" years with vitality and verve. Others endure hot flashes (surges of heat that often strike during the night, making sleeping uncomfortable), insomnia, extra energy, complex emotional duress, weight gain, memory loss, food cravings, endocrine system malfunctions, breast tenderness, spotty bleeding, and vaginal soreness and dryness. These symptoms often mimic those of adrenal insufficiency, which it may very well be, since the adrenal glands pick up where the ovaries left off, producing extra (though possibly sporadic) estrogen hormones. Herbs that nourish the adrenal glands, such as lemon balm and licorice, can help lessen the severity of many menopausal symptoms.

The mainstream medical establishment recommends allopathic estrogen replacement therapy (ERT), which may or may not work and often has side effects. Instead, you need to develop confidence in treating your own body and learning to recognize the difference between an illness and a natural life cycle such as menopause. It's a journey, and instead of canceling the trip, simply put some salve on your blisters and keep walking.

Menopause Friend Tincture

Yields 2 cups

2 teaspoons dried black cohosh (or 5 teaspoons fresh)

2 teaspoons dried chaste tree berries (or 5 teaspoons fresh)

2 teaspoons dried angelica (or 5 teaspoons fresh)

1 teaspoon dried lemon balm (or 3 teaspoons fresh)

1 teaspoon dried mugwort leaves (or 3 teaspoons fresh)

1½ cups grain alcohol (such as vodka or brandy)

½ cup water

2 teaspoons vegetable glycerin (optional)

Wise Women embrace menopause as part of the wonderful journey of life. To ease the symptoms of this third and last of a woman's cycles (maiden, mother, and crone) consider all the women who have gone before you with courage and good spirits, and make the following tincture.

If you like, add any combination of the following herbs to the ingredients already listed: oatstraw, licorice, raspberry leaf, red clover, blue vervain, fenugreek, flaxseed, wild yam, or holy basil. Include marshmallow if vaginal dryness or soreness is a problem and lady's mantle if you're experiencing excess bleeding or spotting.

Follow the instructions in chapter 4: Medicine-Making Methods for making an alcohol tincture. Take it in hot tea or water 2 to 3 times daily, following the dosage guidelines on pages 287–90. Take doses in the morning and afternoon if your symptoms include emotional problems and pelvic congestion, and in the afternoon and evening if you have sleeping problems and hot flashes.

Martha's Vineyard Wise Woman Herbal Tea

This tea blend is a mineral-rich, soothing tonic for the entire nervous system. It's a tasty brew that is high in calcium and magnesium, with an earthy green flavor.

Combine the herbs in a 1-quart glass jar. Pour enough boiling water over them to fill the jar. Stir with a long-handled wooden spoon, and steep for 10 to 15 minutes. (For a brew that's extra rich in minerals, steep the tea overnight and strain it in the morning.) Strain the tea, sweeten to taste, and drink 3 to 4 cups daily. Store the tea in a thermos or jar and refrigerate any leftover tea for up to 24 hours.

Yields 1 quart

2 tablespoons dried nettle leaves
2 tablespoons dried lemon balm
1 teaspoon dried alfalfa
1 teaspoon dried oatstraw
Honey or maple syrup

SEXUAL HEALTH AND LIBIDO

A strong sexual libido requires good nutrition and adequate sleep, along with fun "hints" to your psyche, such as wearing flattering clothing and planning special dates with your partner. The following herbs are revered as nourishing sexual tonics, especially in the Ayurvedic system of herbal medicine. Damiana is admired the world over for its rejuvenating abilities and is prized by both men and women who work long hours or are trekking great distances. Gotu kola is a small violet-like herb with tasty leaves that is used for enhancing memory since it stimulates blood flow to the brain.

Women's Ultimate Tonic Elixir

Yields 1 quart

1 tablespoon cardamom
    seeds

½ teaspoon (8 to 10)
    whole cloves (optional)

1 cup mixture of dried
    dates, apricots, and
    raisins, chopped

3 rounded tablespoons
    dried damiana

3 rounded tablespoons
    dried gotu kola

⅓ cup dried rose petals

2 teaspoons dried blue
    vervain

1 quart fresh water

¼ to ½ cup molasses

½ cup brandy

1 teaspoon vanilla extract

This sweet, delicious, iron-rich tonic can be taken by the tablespoonful or stirred into a bowl of hot oatmeal as an extraordinarily nutrient-rich sweetener. The herbal and fruit sources of iron provide valuable minerals for women with anemia, menorrhagia (heavy menstrual bleeding), and frequent bruising.

Lightly chop together the cardamom seeds, cloves (if using), and dried fruit in a mortar and pestle or a food processor. In a large soup pot, combine this mixture with the rest of the herbs and spices. Cover them with water, stir to blend, and bring the mixture to a boil. Reduce the heat and simmer for 2 to 3 hours, until the water has reduced to about 3 cups. Strain the liquid and pour it into a clean 1-quart glass jar. Add the molasses and stir. Pour in the brandy and vanilla and stir. Store the jar in the refrigerator for up to six months. Take 2 to 3 tablespoons per day.

UTERINE HEALTH

Women of all ages need to address uterine and pelvic health for a variety of reasons. Newly menstruating young women sometimes have extremely heavy periods (menorrhagia), severe menstrual cramping (dysmenorrhea), very irregular cycles, or missing periods (amenorrhea). Congestion in the pelvis can result from stress or from physical causes such as cysts and tumors. To relieve mild congestion and strengthen the uterus in preparation for conception, use the formulas in this section. For extreme blood loss or swelling, consult a health care practitioner immediately. For menstrual cramps, use the Wild Yam PMS Jam in the "Hormones and Premenstrual Syndrome" section.

Wild Raspberry Tonic

Raspberry has, in herbal tradition, an affinity for the pelvic area and is often used to address pelvic congestion and "blockages" in the uterus, ovaries, and pelvis. Use this tonic to nourish the uterus and keep it strong and healthy. (See also chapter 15: Cleansing and Detox.)

Place the raspberry leaves in a 1-quart glass jar. Pour enough boiling water over them to fill the jar, and allow to steep overnight. Strain and gently reheat the liquid to sweeten it, then store it in a thermos and drink 1 to 3 cups daily. Refrigerate any leftover tea for up to 24 hours.

Yields 1 quart

1 ounce (by weight) dried raspberry leaves, chopped or shredded
Maple syrup or honey

Pelvic Toner Tea

This is another option for strengthening and "lightening" the pelvic area when congestion, pain, cramping, irregular menstrual cycles, and stress-induced pelvic and uterine symptoms occur.

Combine all the herbs in a 1-quart glass jar. Pour enough boiling water over them to fill the jar. Steep for 10 to 15 minutes. Strain the tea, sweeten to taste, and store in a thermos. Drink it freely and refrigerate any leftover tea for up to 24 hours.

Yields 1 quart

2 tablespoons dried chaste tree berries
1 tablespoon dried raspberry leaves
1 tablespoon dried spearmint leaves
1 tablespoon dried rose petals

YEAST INFECTIONS

Yeast (*Candida albicans*) is a fungal infection that thrives in moist, dark, and warm places such as the armpits, groin, and vagina. In babies (where it thrives in the mouth), it is called thrush. Yeast infections of the vagina are annoying, extremely itchy, smelly, and wet, leaving underpants soiled and the skin of the labia raw, red, and painful. Many over-the-counter remedies are quite successful at eliminating this fungus; they can also be quite expensive and may or may not work on the first application.

Natural remedies for treating yeast abound, and many ingredients can be found in the home kitchen:

- Garlic is a fabulous antifungal. At the first sign of a yeast infection, peel a clove of garlic and, if desired, wrap it in a bit of cheesecloth or thin cotton fabric. Insert it into the vagina at night and leave it in; use a pantiliner in your underwear. Carefully remove the clove and fabric in the morning. If the garlic produces a burning sensation, leave it in for only 15 to 20 minutes instead of overnight.
- Douche with yogurt, and eat yogurt frequently. Make sure it is unsweetened, unflavored, and contains live probiotic cultures. Train your taste buds to appreciate plain yogurt.
- Avoid alcohol, sugars (refined, brown, and fruit), wheat, and starches. These provide fodder for the parasitic fungus and will prolong the problem.
- Use probiotics that include *Lactobacillus acidophilus*, *L. bulgaricus*, and *L. thermophilus*. They will restore the natural balance of "good" cultures normally found in your gastrointestinal tract, which is especially useful if your yeast infection is a result of taking antibiotic medications.
- Take pau d'arco capsules, 200 to 500 milligrams, daily by mouth.

For more remedies, see chapter 5: For the Expectant and New Mother. For yeast infections associated with eczema or psoriasis, see chapter 15: Cleansing and Detox.

Calendula Suppository

A suppository (bolus) is inserted directly into the vagina (or the rectum for the treatment of hemorrhoids or prostate inflammation). Simple to make, a bolus can be an unusual medicine to create in the kitchen and a great conversation starter when a neighbor stops by and sees you molding long, phallic-shaped rods with your hands. Though the actual application is not fun, it is not unpleasant either, especially when combined with thoughtful care and respectful attention. The soothing results are well worth it.

Yields approximately 60 suppositories

2 cups cocoa butter or coconut oil

2 to 4 teaspoons powdered calendula or other herbs

Follow the instructions in chapter 4: Medicine-Making Methods for making a suppository. Useful herbs for yeast infections include powdered garlic, calendula flowers, witch hazel leaves, goldenseal root, yarrow leaves, Saint-John's-wort flowers, and pau d'arco. Insert a suppository at bedtime and wear a pad or pantiliner in your underwear to catch leaks. Many women find they need to use one suppository each night for a week. Store these suppositories in the refrigerator where they will keep up to one year.

Chapter Eight

ESPECIALLY FOR MEN

Just as many herbs demonstrate a special "affinity" for women, many also work especially well for men. Just like women, men need to find the solitude and quiet time to ground themselves and release extra energy to avoid a buildup of tension in the body. The following formulas address problems of a sexual nature, such as prostate issues and deficient libido, as well as muscle aches and pains.

PROSTATE PROBLEMS

Nearly half of all men over age forty-five suffer some sort of prostate problem, whether mild or benign inflammation; benign prostatic hypertrophy (BPH); or prostate cancer, a leading cause of death among men. Herbs have a rightful place in prostate therapies for both nutritive and supportive functions. Many herbs are anti-inflammatory, diuretic, and demulcent (soothing) and can keep a prostate healthy. Other herbs, especially saw palmetto, are good for reducing the likelihood of prostate cancer and inhibiting cancer precursors.

The following formula can be used proactively (as a preventive measure) and also during treatment for more intense or chronic prostate problems. Consult with your health care practitioner to determine what dosage is right for you.

"Get to the Root of the Problem"
Prostate Tonic 🌿

This root-and-berry tincture is a convenient, concentrated extract of soothing, diuretic, and anti-inflammatory herbs.

Follow the instructions in chapter 4: Medicine-Making Methods for making an alcohol tincture, using grain alcohol such as vodka. If you'd like the tincture to be tastier and more like a cordial, tincture all the herbs but the ginger; make a separate syrup with the ginger, following the instructions in chapter 4: Medicine-Making Methods for making a syrup. Combine the tincture and syrup, and follow the dosage guidelines on pages 287–90.

Yields approximately 1½ cups

3 teaspoons dried saw
   palmetto berries
2 teaspoons fresh yarrow
   leaves
2 teaspoons dried
   marshmallow root,
   chopped
2 teaspoons fresh nettle root
1 teaspoon powdered ginger
½ teaspoon dried turmeric
   root
1 cup vodka
1 cup water

Prostate Suppository 🌿

Although not enjoyable to administer, this suppository is certainly useful for soothing inflamed tissues, cooling burning sensations, shrinking a swollen prostate gland, and easing frequent burning urination. You'll quickly realize the value of a suppository when the tissues are no longer inflamed and sitting and riding become comfortable again.

Follow the instructions in chapter 4: Medicine-Making Methods for making a suppository. Insert the suppository and lie down for 30 to 60 minutes or overnight. Wear a pad or cloth in your underwear to catch leaks. Use each night until symptoms disappear.

*Yields approximately 60
   suppositories*

2 cups cocoa butter or
   coconut oil
2 teaspoons powdered
   saw palmetto berries
1 teaspoon powdered
   marshmallow root
1 teaspoon powdered
   plantain root

SEXUAL HEALTH

Many men's herbals (or sections of women's herbals that instruct on men's health) include powerful and delicious recipes for tonics, but they usually are based on exotic herbs such as astragalus, ashwagandha, fo-ti, damiana, and especially ginseng. In an effort to bring men's herbal health closer to home and to use the Essential Herbs established in this book, the following formulas use common North American herbs and easy-to-find plants without intimidating instructions.

Men's Grounding Formula

Yields 1 cup

2 teaspoons fresh wild
   sarsaparilla root,
   chopped
2 teaspoons fresh
   peppermint
½ teaspoon fresh yarrow
   leaves
½ cup vodka
½ cup water

A grounding tonic, this tincture is specifically formulated to help men support their health and feel more centered. It can be a wonderful supplement for a waning libido or erectile dysfunction simply on the basis of its strength-generating properties. Women can use this formula too when they feel the need for centering and deep strength.

Follow the instructions in chapter 4: Medicine-Making Methods for making an alcohol tincture. Use this formula as a safe, long-term tonic for general sustenance, or take a medicinal dose of 10 to 20 drops twice daily on the tongue or mixed in tea. Drops of this tincture can also be mixed into a teaspoon of Deep Forest Massage Oil just before a massage.

WILD SARSAPARILLA
Aralia nudicaulis

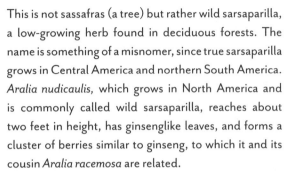

This is not sassafras (a tree) but rather wild sarsaparilla, a low-growing herb found in deciduous forests. The name is something of a misnomer, since true sarsaparilla grows in Central America and northern South America. *Aralia nudicaulis,* which grows in North America and is commonly called wild sarsaparilla, reaches about two feet in height, has ginsenglike leaves, and forms a cluster of berries similar to ginseng, to which it and its cousin *Aralia racemosa* are related.

Wild sarsaparilla root is long and stringy and runs horizontally just under the surface of the ground, growing in colonies on the forest floor. This is an excellent substitute for ginseng, since species of that plant are unfortunately overharvested while wild sarsaparilla is plentiful throughout the northeastern United States. As always, harvest with respect. When a friend and I harvested wild sarsaparilla and first tasted the root tincture, we each felt an immediate grounding effect. I can only describe it as tingling energy traveling from my upper body through my legs to my feet, a very grounding feeling. The effect is immediate and strengthening.

MEN'S EMOTIONAL HEALTH

There is debate about whether men's emotional health is cyclical, like women's, since there is no menstruation. I believe men are just as in tune with the natural rhythms of the world as women are and with the cause and effect of external stressors that create internal disease. Moreover, any kind of stress can create imbalance and illness (for both sexes), for which herbs can provide profound relief. For men, warming herbs are generally chosen, as these are traditionally believed to be more male-oriented, robust, grounding, and strengthening.

Stress-Less Tonic Tea

Yields 1 quart

2 tablespoons dried
  elderberries

2 tablespoons dried wild
  sarsaparilla root

2 tablespoons dried
  peppermint

This tea offers the grounding strength of yang tonic herbs as well as the nervine protection of the Essential Herbs. It has a robust flavor, so you may want to sweeten it with honey. Triple the quantities given here if you're using fresh herbs.

In a 1-quart glass jar, combine the herbs and roots. Pour enough boiling water over them to fill the jar, and stir carefully. Let the tea steep for 30 minutes to 1 hour, then strain. Sweeten the tea as desired and store it in a thermos; drink 3 to 4 cups daily.

Squibnocket Soother

Yields 1 quart

2 tablespoons dried spearmint

2 tablespoons dried lemon
  balm

1 teaspoon dried oatstraw

1 teaspoon dried hops flowers

Affectionately called "Squibby," Squibnocket Beach is a favorite place for Martha's Vineyard families to relax, rejuvenate, and refresh. Similarly, this tea is a nerve-calming tonic infusion with a slightly bitter tang and a refreshing flavor.

In a 1-quart glass jar, combine the herbs and cover them with enough boiling water to fill the jar. Let the tea steep for 5 to 8 minutes. Sweeten it with honey, and drink it before bedtime to ease feelings of stress or anxiety and to experience restful sleep.

Chilmark Chai

Yields 4 to 5 cups

2 tablespoons broken orange pekoe (black) tea

½ teaspoon broken cinnamon sticks

½ teaspoon dried ginger pieces

½ teaspoon nettle herb

⅛ teaspoon pepper

2 whole cloves

When my husband and I lived in Chilmark on Martha's Vineyard, our house was nestled between a rolling meadow, the Atlantic Ocean, and a tiny fishing village. On chilly mornings, we'd sip this hot chai and listen to the sounds of geese overhead, the waves of the ocean, and the sing-song bell of the buoy in the harbor. This is an aromatic, caffeinated black chai with a rich, velvety texture and a lot of peppery spice. The nettle counterbalances the pepper with smoothness and extra minerals.

Combine all ingredients in a teapot and cover them with 1 quart boiling water. Let the tea steep for 4 to 8 minutes. Add sugar and cream to taste, and serve.

BODY CARE FOR MEN

Men's body care needs are generally maintenance-oriented. Assuming you are following a nutritious diet, getting adequate sleep, and keeping a positive attitude, the following formulas will help maintain skin and muscle health and will indirectly strengthen cardiovascular and emotional health.

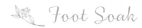

Deep Forest Massage Oil

Yields 1 cup

1 cup sweet almond oil

20 drops balsam fir
essential oil

10 drops birch essential oil

5 drops wintergreen
essential oil

5 drops ginger essential oil

1 vitamin E capsule,
optional

This is a luxurious oil for easing sore muscles, promoting relaxation, stimulating blood circulation, and encouraging overall enjoyment.

Whisk the oils together in a glass bowl. Break open the vitamin E capsule, if using, and squeeze the contents into the oil. Whisk together and store the mixture in a glass jar with a tight-fitting lid. During a massage, allow the oil to warm in the palms of your hands before applying it to the skin.

The oil has a shelf life of approximately six to twelve months.

Foot Soak

Yields 1 quart

1 tablespoon dried yarrow

1 tablespoon powdered
ginger

2 to 3 whole cloves

2 tablespoons Dead Sea
salts

This quick and easy preparation warms sore feet, stimulates blood flow, and soothes these extremities that bear so much weight.

Combine the herbs with the salts in a large soup pot. Pour 4 cups boiling water over them and steep for 10 to 15 minutes. Carefully strain and reserve the liquid, and pour it into a glass or ceramic bowl or back into the cleaned soup pot. Sit down and soak your feet in this very warm tea for 10 to 20 minutes.

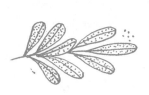

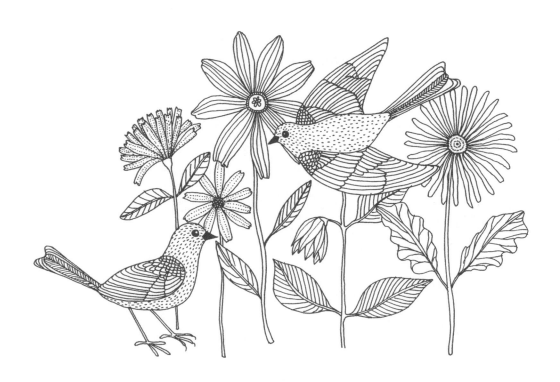

Part Four

RECIPES AND REMEDIES FOR HEALTHY LIVING

Healing is a matter of time, but it is sometimes also a matter of opportunity.

—Hippocrates

The most beautiful experience, the most enriching, is the love that the plants have taught me. Because to care for another is to love one's neighbor. Attend his suffering and restore the joy of living. Restore health, the most essential thing in life.

—Grandmother Bernadette Rébiénot

Chapter Nine

—◦✎◦—

EVERYDAY TONICS FOR VITALITY

We all need our daily boost of nourishing vitamins and minerals, amino acids, probiotic cultures, and other sustaining and body-building nutrients. Usually we get these through our diet, as most food contains a perfect combination to suit our bodies' needs. But sometimes we don't eat properly or eat the wrong amounts. Or our immune system may be out of balance because of illness or stress, so the foods we eat don't nourish us as optimally as they should. Herbal medicine excels in these situations because of the tonic properties of herbs.

VITAMIN C AND IMMUNITY

Many herbs come replete with all the nutrients we need, if only we consume them in the proper quantities. Often, this means taking them as teas, since we replenish water-based vitamins in our bodies when we drink teas. The body can more easily process the nutrients it gets throughout the day from several cups of tea than those delivered all at once in a pill or capsule.

The following tonics are meant to supplement a wholesome, balanced diet. If used consistently, they will provide vitality in the form of better energy, a more positive outlook, a feeling of being in shape, glowing skin, shiny hair, and better endurance.

Vitamin C–Rose Hip Decoction

Yields 3 cups

2 cups dried rose hips

3 cups water

Vitamin C is easy to come by: it's in guavas, oranges, grapefruit, strawberries, kiwis, red and green bell peppers, brussels sprouts, and melons such as cantaloupe. It's also extremely high in rose hips; dried rose hips contain nearly 2,000 milligrams per 100 grams of hips, whereas oranges contain only 45 milligrams per 100 grams of orange. The recommended daily allowance of vitamin C is 90 milligrams for men and 75 milligrams for women.

Rub the rose hips in a tea towel to remove the tiny hairs and bristles. Put them in a saucepan and cover them with the water. Bring to a boil, then reduce the heat and simmer, tightly covered, for 15 to 20 minutes. The decoction will taste very tart. Sweeten as desired (diluting it with apple juice is a delicious balancing option), and drink 1 to 3 cups daily.

HERBAL SOURCES OF VITAMIN C

The following herbs and uncommon fruits are high in vitamin C; use them in your meals daily for an added boost during the winter. Fresh herbs contain the highest concentration of vitamins.

Amla saar (Indian gooseberry)	Mustard greens
Chickweed	Black currant
Dandelion	Rose hips

Cooking spices and herbs rich in vitamin C include oregano, chili pepper, basil, cayenne pepper, cloves, fennel, and parsley.

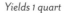
The four herbs in this recipe combine well to create immune-boosting infusions, syrups, or tinctures. I recommend infusions for long-term tonics that will be used for weeks or months at a time. Other immune-boosting herbs to supplement these four include echinacea, astragalus, olive leaf, and garlic.

As a Tea

Yields 1 quart

Using a 1-quart jar, follow the instructions in chapter 4: Medicine-Making Methods for making an herbal infusion. Drink 1 to 3 cups daily.

2 tablespoons dried red clover

2 tablespoons dried peppermint

2 tablespoons dried elderberries

¼ teaspoon powdered ginger

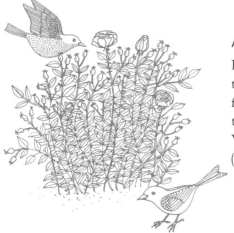

As a Syrup

Yields 2 cups

Follow the instructions in chapter 4: Medicine-Making Methods for making a syrup. Take 1 to 3 teaspoons daily, preferably in the Vitamin C–Rose Hip Decoction (described earlier in this section).

2 tablespoons dried red clover

2 tablespoons dried peppermint

2 tablespoons dried elderberries

2 tablespoons fresh ginger, chopped

½ cup fresh red clover

¼ cup fresh peppermint

¼ cup fresh elderberries

2 tablespoons fresh ginger, chopped

2 cups vodka

1 cup vegetable glycerin

1 cup water

As a Tincture

Follow the instructions in chapter 4: Medicine-Making Methods for making an alcohol tincture. Take ½ teaspoon 3 times daily for three or more weeks.

ENERGY

The best avenue toward consistent energy is a healthy diet, regular exercise, adequate sleep, a positive attitude, and a good sense of humor. Caffeine-containing teas, coffee, and chocolate give you a quick boost, but they come with drawbacks such as headaches or extreme lethargy once the caffeine wears off. They can also affect your appetite and be addictive.

For long-term energy, I prefer herbs that are safe and sustaining. Their plant chemicals stimulate the body to perform, give a feeling of aliveness, lift the spirits, and wake you up. All this without caffeine!

Many people use ginseng for increasing energy, as it can have a sharp, caffeinelike effect. But because the *Panax* ginsengs are at risk and have been overharvested for centuries, I've never used them. I've also been told by the ginseng that it is not a plant for me, and after living in the rich Appalachian mountains and rarely finding wild ginseng, I believe it probably isn't the plant for many other people either. Thankfully, there are other valuable and wonderful herbs that stimulate vitality, energy, memory function, and verve.

Damiana is an herb of rejuvenation, long revered in Ayurvedic and Asian medicine as a restorative. Also prized as a sexual tonic for both men and women, damiana is a nervine tonic and strengthener. Gotu kola is a small tropical herb known as a tonic for the nerves and an "antidote" to memory loss. Often paired with ginkgo, it stimulates blood flow to the brain. Astragalus is used as a long-term immune booster, and the fruits are antioxidant.

Energy Elixir

This powerful and delicious elixir is really a syrup preserved with brandy. This is a potent way to make a long-lasting tonic.

Combine all the herbs in a pot and pour the boiling water over them. Steep, loosely covered, for 1 hour, or until the liquid is reduced by about half. Strain, and pour the liquid into a 1-quart glass jar. Allow it to cool, then add the sweetener and brandy. Take 1 to 2 tablespoons per day for energy. Stored in the refrigerator, this elixir's shelf life is approximately six months.

Yields 1 quart

2 tablespoons dried damiana
2 tablespoons dried gotu kola
1 tablespoon dried astragalus
1 tablespoon dried black cherry
1 tablespoon dried licorice
1 tablespoon dried elderberries
4 cups boiling water
½ cup sugar, honey, or vegetable glycerin
½ cup brandy

Everyday Tonic for Vitality and Vigor

The herbs in this tonic combine well because they are so nutritive, and this easy nutrition provides long-term energy. This formula can be taken as a tea, syrup, or tincture, using the same herbs in the same proportions. I recommend infusions for long-term tonics.

As a Tea

Follow the instructions in chapter 4: Medicine-Making Methods for making an herbal infusion. Drink 1 to 3 cups daily. Though it's not necessary, you may wish to prepare the dandelion root and leaves separately, making a decoction with the roots and an infusion with the leaves. You can then combine them and sweeten as desired.

Yields 1 quart

2 tablespoons dried spearmint or peppermint
2 tablespoons dried nettle
2 tablespoons dried dandelion root and/or leaves

Yields 2 cups

As a Syrup

Follow the instructions in chapter 4: Medicine-Making Methods for making a syrup. Take 1 to 3 teaspoons daily, preferably in Wild Herbflower Tea (see chapter 7: Especially for Women) or Women's Everyday Tonic Tea (described later in this section).

⅓ cup dried spearmint or
    peppermint
⅓ cup dried nettle
⅓ cup dried dandelion
    root and/or leaves
½ cup sugar or honey

Yields 4 cups

As a Tincture

Using a 1-quart jar, follow the instructions in chapter 4: Medicine-Making Methods for making an alcohol tincture. Take ½ teaspoon 3 times daily.

1 cup fresh spearmint or
    peppermint
1 cup fresh nettle
1 cup fresh dandelion root
    and/or leaves
2 cups vodka or brandy
1 cup vegetable glycerin
1 cup water

Vinegar-and-Honey Oxymel

Yields 2½ to 3 cups

Sometimes called an elixir, an oxymel is simply an acid-and-sugar preparation that is usually made with honey and vinegar. It can be an effective agent for taking energy herbs such as damiana, gotu kola, ashwaghanda, or rose hips, or for bitter or strong-tasting herbs such as motherwort and garlic.

1 to 2 cups honey
1 cup apple cider vinegar
Fresh or dried
    damiana, gotu kola,
    ashwaghanda, and/or
    rose hips, chopped

Follow the instructions in chapter 4: Medicine-Making Methods, under "Honey-Based Medicines," for making an oxymel. Store in the pantry and take 1 teaspoon 2 to 3 times daily if you're using energy herbs.

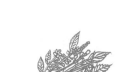

A nourishing tonic infusion for wellness and vitality. Sustaining, mineralizing, and balancing for both young men and women. Delicious!

Using a 1-quart glass jar, combine the herbs and pour enough boiling water over them to fill the jar. Steep for 5 to 8 minutes or overnight. Strain the tea well and drink it freely.

Yields 1 quart

1 tablespoon dried nettle
   leaves
1 tablespoon dried gotu
   kola
1 tablespoon dried lemon
   balm
1 teaspoon dried alfalfa
½ teaspoon dried rose
   hips, chopped

Women's Everyday Tonic Tea

Tonic is an herbalist's word for an herb that can safely be used long-term with maximum nourishment. Certain herbs often act as tonics on particular body systems; for instance, in this formula, raspberry is a uterine and pelvic tonic, lemon balm is a nervous system tonic, and red clover and nettle are skeletal system tonics.

Using a 1-quart glass jar, follow the instructions in chapter 4: Medicine-Making Methods for making an herbal infusion. Strain the tea well and drink it freely.

Yields 1 quart

2 tablespoons dried red
   clover
2 tablespoons dried nettle
2 tablespoons dried lemon
   balm
1 teaspoon dried rose
   petals
1 teaspoon dried raspberry
   leaves

Chapter Ten

SNIFFLES, COLDS, AND VIRUSES

No matter how many times we scrub the house, wash our hands, or bundle up in bad weather, we are all susceptible to colds and influenza. Germs and viruses have adapted alongside humanity for thousands of years, but fortunately, many helpful edible and medicinal plants have adapted with us too. From this wealth of green life, we can use those that will not only relieve the symptoms of colds and flu but also provide a holistic approach for the care of many body systems at once. These healing herbs both nourish the spirit and fight disease.

For children, start with smaller amounts of herbal remedies (use the dosage guidelines on pages 287–90) and use a variety of healing aids. For instance, most children are sensitive enough to respond positively to extra sleep. Include extra liquids in their diet as well as fresh herbs in their food and medicine.

Children and sensitive adults often respond well to liquids administered topically. A warm compress soaked in tea and placed on the belly, chest, or forehead is an easy way to administer medicine to an infant or young child. A foot soak or wrap in a strong, hot tea can also be a soothing way to give your child medicine, since the skin on the feet readily absorbs certain plant chemicals. This is a great method for administering ginger or peppermint if your child is vomiting or has an upset stomach and cannot keep liquids down.

Be sure to remove dairy from the diet during colds and flu for both children and adults. Other potential dietary allergens include wheat, eggs, corn, and soy, and each should be avoided or eaten in scant amounts while the body is healing.

COUGHS

Coughing is the body's way of removing particulates from the lungs, and there's more to it than just expelling air. The lower bronchioles create phlegm, a mucouslike substance that lubricates the lungs and can be coughed up. The cough spasm can be painful, and the throat may become irritated and inflamed.

Dry coughs are annoying because they seem to do nothing, yet they are persistent and irritating to the sinus and throat tissues. Chronic conditions such as bronchitis can benefit from the following treatment along with other natural therapies such as hot showers; warm, moist rooms (use a humidifier); plenty of warm liquids; eucalyptus chest rubs (see Eucalyptus-Menthol Respiratory Salve in chapter 6: For Infant and Child); and extra garlic and cayenne pepper, two of my favorite remedies.

Dry Cough Tea

A cough that is hacking, dry, and shallow is of no use. It's simply the muscles around the lungs convulsing because of triggers within the lungs and throat, but without excretory mucous in the lungs, the cough accomplishes nothing. The herbs in this tea are antispasmodic, soothing, and expectorant.

Combine the herbs in a 1-quart glass jar, and cover them with enough boiling water to fill the jar. Cap the jar and steep for 8 to 12 minutes, or to desired strength. Strain the tea well (it will be rather thick) and store in a thermos. Drink it hot, ½ cup every 30 minutes until symptoms subside.

Yields 1 quart

2 tablespoons dried
　marshmallow root
2 tablespoons dried
　licorice root
1 tablespoon dried coltsfoot
1 teaspoon dried anise

Wet Cough Tea

Yields 1 quart

2 tablespoons dried
  elderberries
2 tablespoons dried sage
2 tablespoons dried thyme
Honey
Fresh lemon juice

Wet coughs are generally productive (expelling mucous), which is the body's way of removing unwanted substances. However, some wet coughs can become explosive and overwhelming. The herbs in this tea help calm and partly dry out an overly wet cough. Thyme is a powerful upper and lower respiratory antibacterial herb.

Combine the herbs in a 1-quart glass jar. Pour enough boiling water over them to fill the jar. Steep for 5 to 8 minutes, tightly covered. Strain the tea, and add honey and fresh lemon juice to taste. Store it hot in a thermos, and drink 3 to 5 cups daily.

Wild Weed Cough Brew

Yields 1 quart

2 tablespoons dried
  licorice root
1 tablespoon dried
  marshmallow root
1 tablespoon dried mullein
  leaves
1 tablespoon dried plantain
  leaves
1 tablespoon dried violet
  leaves
1 teaspoon dried ginger (or
  ¼ teaspoon powdered)
Honey (optional)

These herbs make a wonderful cough infusion to help with general coughs, muscle aches, and lower respiratory congestion.

Combine the herbs in a 1-quart glass jar and cover with enough boiling water to fill the jar. Steep for 15 to 30 minutes, tightly covered. Strain the tea, add honey if desired, and store it in a hot thermos. Drink ½ cup every 30 minutes, up to 4 cups a day.

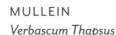

MULLEIN
Verbascum Thapsus

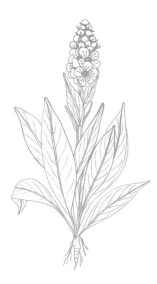

Mullein is a distinctly recognizable plant, with a tall stalk that rises up to six feet and huge, velvety, fuzzy leaves at the base that taper into smaller leaves higher up. Its flowers are pea-sized and bright yellow, growing on a fuzzy, coblike spike. For centuries, mullein leaves have been prized for treating respiratory ailments, particularly bronchitis. The leaves are high in mucilage (like plantain) and will soothe hard, painful, and chronic coughs. The plant is also useful as a tea for convalescent periods when you are recovering from a long spell of coughing (such as with bronchitis, pneumonia, or whooping cough). In the past, native peoples of the Americas smoked mullein leaves, inhaling the beneficial and soothing smoke directly into inflamed bronchial membranes.

A favorite herbal remedy for earache involves gently heating mullein flowers in oil that is dropped into the ear canal. This may originate from an old German practice mentioned by herbal historian Alma Hutchens, whereby the mullein was used to treat deafness. Topically, mullein leaves make a good addition to salves and oils. Since they dry well, they can be kept on hand throughout the winter for use as needed.

Kitchen Cough Elixir

Yields 1 to 2 cups

This is an easy, on-the-fly herbal honey for treating stubborn and acute coughs.

1 onion, chopped

3 cloves garlic, chopped

1 1-inch piece fresh ginger, chopped

1 1-inch piece cinnamon stick

1 to 2 cups honey

The night before you want to use the elixir, chop the vegetables and herbs and place them in a stainless steel pot or a ceramic or glass bowl. Pour enough honey over the herbs to submerge them and stir. Cover the pot or bowl with a lid or plastic wrap, and allow the mixture to stand overnight.

In the morning, strain off the honey with its accumulated juices, stir to blend, and bottle them together, storing the bottle in a pantry or cabinet. Do not refrigerate. Take 1 to 2 teaspoons every other hour as needed. This elixir will keep up to six months.

Elderberry-Currant Honey

Yields 2 cups

Many wild fruits ease bronchial spasms and coughs. Beloved gypsy herbalist Juliette de Bairacli Levy recommends wild currants, and many herbalists prize elderberry.

1 cup black currants

1 cup elderberries

2 cups honey

Pound the berries in a stainless steel pot, and pour the honey over them. Bring the mixture to a gentle simmer over low heat. Maintain the simmer for 10 to 20 minutes. Strain the solids, bottle the honey and the accumulated juices, and take 1 to 2 teaspoons every other hour as needed. Stored in the pantry or cabinet, this will keep up to six months.

LOW IMMUNITY

The immune system is an intricate and highly functional garden that includes the lymph system, digestive system, circulatory system, waste removal system, and even muscular and nervous systems. Think about it:

when we succumb to a cold, we feel sluggish and our thought processes aren't as sharp. Even our muscles ache. This is a perfect time to address the body holistically.

We cannot expect to pop a pill from the store and experience instant wellness. The body requires sustenance and care, and we can easily provide this with natural—and even pleasant—remedies.

You have a wealth of resources to call on when caring for those with colds and flu. Herbs lend themselves readily to crafting homemade remedies, and most of these can be created in minutes. Especially if a garden is accessible, you should be able to use these recipes for quick relief in a pinch, or you can put the ingredients together beforehand so these useful formulas are ready throughout the year.

West Chop Winter Tea for Colds and Flu

This formula contains herbs that stimulate the immune system. Echinacea is a powerhouse of plant chemicals that are antimicrobial, antifungal, antibacterial, and even antistaphylococcal. Cream-colored elder flowers ease catarrh (irritation of mucous membranes) and sinus inflammation, and together with yarrow, they are considered premier fever-reducing herbs. Rose hips are high in vitamin C, spearmint is an excellent circulatory stimulant and nervous system balancer, and licorice is hailed in Chinese medicine as a rejuvenating herb and a remedy for coughs and bronchial irritations. By gathering most of these herbs yourself and purchasing the echinacea, licorice, and astragalus, you can brew a quart of fresh tea for pennies.

On Martha's Vineyard, the two areas that flank the main harbor are referred to as East Chop and West Chop. In the summer, these sunny neighborhoods are witness to hundreds of sailing vessels from all over the world; in the winter, they are gray, bleak, and incredibly windy. We occasionally take a family drive up the chops in the dead of winter to watch the fierce Nantucket

Yields 1 quart

2 tablespoons dried lemon balm leaves

2 tablespoons dried spearmint leaves

1 tablespoon dried elderberries

1 teaspoon dried echinacea root, chopped

1 teaspoon dried elder flowers

1 teaspoon licorice root, chopped

1 teaspoon mullein leaves

1 teaspoon dried rose hips

(cont.)

Optional bitter herbs:

1 teaspoon astragalus root, chopped

½ teaspoon wild cherry bark

½ teaspoon white willow bark

½ teaspoon yarrow leaves or flowers

Honey

Sound's waves smashing against the shore; there's never traffic. My children ask for West Chop Winter Tea at the first sign of feeling poorly. They like that it's a delicious hot tea with a slightly bitter taste and is easily blended with honey. The combination of herbs is open to experimentation; feel free to include the optional ones that resonate with you or are most available in your area.

Combine the herbs in a 1-quart glass jar. Pour enough boiling water over them to fill the jar. Stir, cover the jar, and steep for 20 to 30 minutes. Strain the tea, sweeten to taste, and store it in a large thermos. At the first signs of a cold or flu, drink 2 to 4 cups daily. During colds and flu, drink up to 5 hot cups daily, and plan to make one to two batches per day.

Garlic-Cayenne Juice

Yields 1 cup

1 to 2 cloves raw garlic, finely minced

Dash cayenne pepper (or as much as you can stand)

1 cup grapefruit juice, orange juice, or apple cider

I became a big believer in this potent combination of herbs after my husband introduced me to it. It's simple, quick, and not bad tasting. I often get rid of any hint of cold or flu if I take this juice at the first sign of feeling ill. Even the children will try it; for their sake (and your own) be sure to mince the garlic finely and start with small amounts of cayenne.

Raw garlic (Allium sativum) is a potent antimicrobial, antiviral, antiseptic, and antiparasitic root with a volatile oil that is useful in treating bronchitis, catarrh, asthma, colds, and flu. I consider it an essential food to be eaten daily. Cayenne pepper (Capsicum minimum) is a stimulating diaphoretic; a little goes a long way in stimulating the circulatory system (through both internal and external applications). For our purposes here, it encourages the respiratory system to expel mucous and opens up the airways.

Combine all the ingredients in a ½ pint jar with a lid and shake well. Grapefruit juice does the best job of masking cayenne's heat. Use as much pepper as you can stand and try to drink it all at once. Additional ingredients to try include vitamin C–rich lemon peel and nutritious spirulina. Children may experience an upset tummy after consuming too much cayenne pepper; start with tiny amounts and simply follow each dose with bread or crackers.

Elderberry-Ginger Syrup for Colds and Flu

Syrups are a wonderful way to administer herbs, especially to children, but I admit to being partial to syrups even as an adult. I like to take them by the spoonful and also use them to sweeten my tea. I use them on pancakes and waffles—simply mix equal parts herbal syrup and maple syrup, and you have a tasty and nutritious breakfast treat.

This syrup is a version of my medicinal syrup that won first place for tinctures and extracts at the International Herb Symposium 2007. I've scaled it down to a handful of Essential Herbs that should be easy to get from a field, garden, or local health food store. You might also include yarrow, peppermint, and echinacea.

Follow the instructions in chapter 4: Medicine-Making Methods for making a syrup. Adults should take 1 tablespoon every hour; children should take 2 teaspoons every hour until coughing subsides. For general cold and flu symptoms, adults take 2 to 3 tablespoons daily, children 4 to 6 teaspoons daily.

Yields 2 cups

2 tablespoons fresh elderberries

2 tablespoons fresh lemon balm leaves

2 tablespoons fresh ginger, chopped (skin included)

2 tablespoons fresh red clover blossoms

2 cups honey

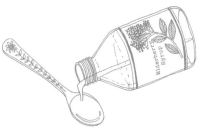

Children's Fever Friend

Yields 1 cup

¼ cup dried elder flowers

¼ cup fresh ginger,
   chopped (or 1 teaspoon
   powdered)

½ cup vegetable glycerin
   or honey

2 teaspoons brandy

½ cup wate

Centuries ago, herbalists used these same herbs to treat their children's fevers, and the efficacy and safety of these plants is why they are still favorite treatments today. If your children love gingery cookies, they'll love this fragrant, thick elixir.

Follow the instructions in chapter 4: Medicine-Making Methods for making a glycerin tincture, using a 1-pint glass jar in place of the 1-quart jar. Administer according to the dosage guidelines on pages 287–90.

Lip-Smacking Tongue Zinger Tincture

Yields 1 cup

¼ cup fresh echinacea
   root, chopped

¼ cup fresh spilanthes
   leaves, chopped

¼ cup fresh raspberries
   (optional)

1 teaspoon lemon juice

¾ cup brandy or vodka

¼ cup water

Immunity-building echinacea can be lots of fun for adventurous children who marvel at the numbing qualities of the root. Simply place a few drops on the tongue and wait for the zingy, numbing sensation to begin. Spilanthes leaves also offer this fun effect; be sure to warn children before dosing them so they aren't surprised and scared at what they're feeling!

Combine the herbs and fruit in a 1-quart glass jar. Follow the instructions in chapter 4: Medicine-Making Methods for making an alcohol tincture. Use the dosage guidelines on pages 287–90 to administer the remedy.

NASAL CONGESTION

The causes of nasal and sinus (upper respiratory) congestion can be many. Environmental allergens such as mites, dust, mold, and pollen are key contributors. Food allergies are also high on the list, and diet should be suspected any time you have sinus congestion. Many people with allergies experience added relief using liver-strengthening and waste removal herbs such as yellow dock and dandelion (see chapter 15: Cleansing and Detox).

Adding fluids to your diet is essential, as extra water helps all body systems operate at peak efficiency. You can put a hot water bottle, well wrapped in a cloth, on your head while resting; this can open up clogged sinus passageways and relieve tightness. A hot shower can also help, especially when using peppermint or rosemary soap or shampoo.

Many herbs are associated with relieving sinus congestion, including bayberry bark, goldenseal root, and horseradish. Bayberry is not easy for many people to find, and goldenseal is on the United Plant Savers' At-Risk list. Horseradish makes a wonderful sinus opener, but its effects are short-lived, and its alarming spiciness is not appreciated—to put it mildly—by small children. In the following remedy, I've used effective Essential Herbs for safety and availability.

Herbalists' Sniffle Friend

This is a gentle, safe formula for children and adults of all ages. The elder flower helps clear sinus passages, the raspberry is mildly astringent, and the lemon balm is nervine to help you relax and tends to move your body's energy to your head—exactly where you want these herbs to go.

Yields 2 cups

2 teaspoons dried elder
   flowers
2 teaspoons dried lemon balm
1 teaspoon dried raspberry
   leaves
2 cups boiling water

As a Tea

Combine the herbs in a teapot and cover them with the water. Steep for 8 to 10 minutes; strain the tea. Drink ¼ cup at a time, as hot as you can tolerate, every 30 minutes, until symptoms subside.

Yields 2 cups

1 tablespoon dried elder
   flowers
1 tablespoon dried lemon
   balm
1 tablespoon dried
   raspberry leaves
2 cups water

For a Compress

Combine the herbs in a 1-quart glass jar and cover them with the water. Steep for 8 to 10 minutes. Strain and reserve the liquid. Soak a soft, clean cloth in the liquid, wring it gently so it won't drip, and place it on the forehead for as long as it stays warm. You can also lay the compress gently across your cheeks and nose; just make sure to keep your nostrils unobstructed.

As a Tincture

Follow the instructions in chapter 4: Medicine-Making Methods for making an alcohol tincture. Use the dosage guidelines on pages 287–90 for infants and children.

Yields 2 cups

1 cup fresh elder flowers

1 cup fresh lemon balm, chopped

¼ cup fresh raspberry leaves, chopped

1 cup brandy

1 cup water

HAY FEVER

Occasionally sinus congestion is caused by pollutants in the environment, such as grass, flower, or tree pollens; dust; mites; molds; or animal fur or cat dander. Poor goldenrod gets blamed as the culprit much of the time, but in fact, many plants produce sinus-clogging pollens, and many more airborne pollutants can interfere with our healthy breathing than we would like to admit. In fact, goldenrod taken as a tea or tincture is a remedy for catarrh and upper respiratory congestion.

Hay fever typically presents with severe upper respiratory symptoms: nasal congestion or nasal fluidity—or sometimes both at the same time. The sinus cavities behind the cheeks can feel clogged like cement blocks, while the lower portion of the nose drips uncontrollably. The eyes water, salivation increases, and headaches often persist.

Many herbs act as drying agents to the mucosal tissues. For the sinuses, goldenseal is one of the best, but we won't use it here for several reasons: it has been overharvested (it's on the United Plant Savers' At-Risk List) and has proven difficult to grow organically. Also, it can be overly drying, to the point that it dries up not only sinus secretions but everything else too. I once took powdered goldenseal root to counter my hay fever while I was nursing my young son. To my surprise, my breast milk promptly dried up. Don't underestimate the power of herbs nor the interconnectedness of the body's systems. Thankfully, other herbs are equally effective, more common, and much safer.

Nettle, or stinging nettle (*Urtica dioica*), is a favorite for treating hay fever. It is nourishing, high in vitamins and minerals, and is so safe that it is a prized food source. For hay fever, it can be taken dried as a tea, though it's often most effective in the form of freeze-dried capsules, which can be found at your local health food store.

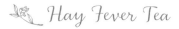

Hay Fever Tea

Yields 1 quart

3 tablespoons dried nettle leaves

3 tablespoons dried elder flowers

1 quart boiling water

This is a mild and delicious infusion of Essential Herbs, and when taken consistently over the course of several days, it can have a significant impact on the misery of hay fever.

Place the herbs in a teapot and cover them with the water. Steep for 10 to 12 minutes; strain the tea and sweeten if desired. Store in a thermos and drink it frequently throughout the day.

SINUSITIS

Chronic sinus congestion can be a sign of a deeper or more serious condition. During a cold, the nasal passageways will sometimes become clogged with polyps or dense mucosal material. This is an indication that there is an imbalance in the body's systems, including the waste removal system. It may also indicate a severe reaction to a certain food substance, so pay attention to your diet and remove wheat, soy, corn, dairy, eggs, and other possible allergens to determine if your sinusitis is a food allergy reaction.

Minty Steam Inhalation

Steam inhalations ease sinusitis and bronchitis. For children, this method can be a challenge, as they may want to open their eyes; join your child under the towel to help him master the process.

Fill a wide-rimmed bowl with steaming hot water and drop in the fresh herbs or essential oil. Lean over the bowl, pull a towel over your head, and inhale, being certain not to open your eyes. Try to breathe through your nose (for sinusitis) or deeply into your lungs (for bronchitis). Use this time under the towel to relax, rub your neck, stretch your shoulders, and massage your scalp. Listen to music or visualize the fragrance of the herbs flowing freely through your respiratory system. Add more hot water as needed and remain under the towel for 5 to 10 minutes at a time; take a break for 10 minutes and repeat. Drink a large glass of room-temperature water afterward.

Yields 1 quart

1 cup fresh peppermint or
  rosemary, chopped;
  or 3 drops mint or
  rosemary essential oil

Elder-Violet Tea

When I lived in the lush mountains of eastern Tennessee, I would often walk out into my garden after a light spring rain to find an entire carpet of blooming purple violets. I could gather basketsful in just a few minutes, and my young children and I would nibble them fresh, eat them in salads, and tuck them behind our ears because they were so beautiful. Elder and violet flowers are delicate blossoms that quickly yield their pro-respiratory properties to boiling water.

Combine the herbs in a 1-quart glass jar and pour enough boiling water over them to fill the jar. Steep for 5 to 8 minutes, tightly covered. Strain the tea, sweeten with honey to taste, and store it in a thermos. Drink 3 cups daily.

Yields 1 quart

2 tablespoons dried elder
  flowers (or 1 cup fresh)
2 tablespoons dried violet
  flowers (or 1 cup fresh)
1 tablespoon dried violet
  leaves (or 1/3 cup fresh)
Honey

EAR INFECTION/EARACHE

See the Mullein Flower Ear Oil in chapter 6: For Infant and Child.

VIRAL INFECTIONS

Some herbs and their essential oils have the scientifically proven capacity to kill viruses, while others stimulate our own immune response against pathogens. Garlic, thyme, and eucalyptus are high in chemicals that can actually kill dangerous microorganisms such as parasites, bacteria, and even some viruses. Lemon balm, Saint-John's-wort, echinacea, and possibly astragalus work to inhibit the action of viral invaders and render them less successful. For instance, echinacea possesses a myriad of phytochemicals that will kill or otherwise help the body resist staphylococcus infections, viral infections, parasites, and bacteria. Herbalists strive to strengthen the body and support its efforts at regaining balance. They employ a variety of herbs to assist, support, strengthen, balance, and revitalize the body and its immune system—and then, yes, to attack the virus.

Lemony Antiviral Tea

Yields 1 quart

3 tablespoons dried lemon
  balm
2 tablespoons dried Saint-
  John's-wort leaves and
  flowers
1 teaspoon dried thyme
Slice of fresh lemon
  (optional)
Honey

The three herbs in this tea are considered antiviral, meaning they either kill the virus or help the body in its efforts to do so. The infusion of these herbs naturally includes their essential oils as well as other phytochemicals that strengthen the body's antiviral efforts.

Combine the herbs in a 1-quart glass jar. Pour enough boiling water over them to fill the jar. Steep for 8 to 10 minutes, tightly covered. Strain the liquid, squeeze in the juice from the lemon slice if desired, and add honey to taste. Store the hot tea in a thermos and drink ½ to 1 cup every hour.

Antiviral Tincture

A tincture is a convenient and concentrated form for taking valuable plant medicines. Fresh herbs are usually used and are more potent in tincture recipes. Take the remedy at the onset of a viral infection, and use it consistently until the infection is completely gone.

Follow the instructions in chapter 4: Medicine-Making Methods for making an alcohol tincture. Use the dosage guidelines on pages 287–90.

Yields 3 to 4 cups

½ cup fresh lemon balm
½ cup fresh echinacea
  root, chopped
¼ cup fresh elderberries
¼ cup fresh elder flowers
¼ cup fresh ginger,
  chopped
¼ cup fresh red clover
2 cups vodka or brandy
1 cup vegetable glycerin
1 cup water

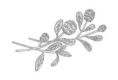

Strengthening Smoothie

Tasty and satisfying, this drink contains the Essential Herbs lemon balm and ginger, which are antiviral, as well as nourishing fruits and probiotic yogurt—a good blend when you are recuperating from a lingering viral infection.

Place the lemon balm and ginger in a stainless steel pot or a teapot, and pour the water over them. Steep for 7 to 8 minutes, tightly covered. Strain the mixture and chill in the refrigerator. Place the frozen fruit (such as bananas, strawberries, grapes, or mangoes) and fruit juice (such as apple, pear, plum, cranberry, pineapple, or orange) in a blender and blend until smooth. Add the chilled herbal tea and yogurt to your preferred consistency.

Yields 3 to 4 cups

2 tablespoons fresh lemon
  balm, chopped
1 tablespoon fresh ginger,
  minced
2 cups boiling water
2 cups frozen fruit
½ cup fruit juice
2 tablespoons yogurt

Chapter Eleven

HEALING WOUNDS

The skin, with all its folds and contours and crevasses and hills, is the body's largest organ and our first line of defense. As such, it is responsible for a wide range of duties: protecting the flesh, keeping out germs and foreign objects, holding in moisture, and acting as a conduit to supply the extremities with fresh blood and oxygen. Our job, as body owners, is to keep our skin clean, clear (and that means clear of soapy detergent residue too), and hydrated so it can function properly.

A healthy diet of fresh grains, vegetables, fruits, and plenty of fresh water will accomplish a great deal of this. Don't smoke; don't use heavy detergents and chemical-laden shampoos and soaps, and use makeup sparingly, if at all. The natural look is a far better option than painted faces that ultimately end up in wrinkles and damaged skin.

The skin receives the brunt of the body's contact with the world, and it often shows. Here are natural, herbal solutions to leave your skin feeling soft, supple, fresh, and strong. Additional remedies can be found in chapter 17: Beauty, Skin, and Body Care.

WOUNDS AND INJURIES

Wound-healing herbs are called vulneraries. If you get hurt, you are vulnerable, and herbs such as yarrow, plantain, comfrey, rosemary, and calendula address common injuries. For example, comfrey's Latin name is *Symphytum*, which derives from the same root as *symphony*. This alludes to its wonderful ability to bring skin tissues together like a symphony.

Use the following ointments and compress to repair broken tissue and heal contusions, rashes, scrapes, cuts, lacerations, burns and sunburns, and infections. Many of the herbs used are antibacterial and antifungal, so they protect against microbial invaders and fight any existing infection, especially when aided by concentrated essential oils. Clove oil is slightly numbing, which can be useful for painful bruises and cuts, and both clove and rosemary are highly antiseptic.

Rosemary's Blessing First Aid Ointment

By far the most successful herbal treatment I've used for external wounds and injuries, this is my business' best-selling first aid ointment. It's a combination of common yard "weeds" with a few woodland herbs thrown in, and it never fails to restore health, elasticity, and smoothness to skin that's been damaged or cut. Use fresh but lightly wilted herbs.

Follow the instructions in chapter 4: Medicine-Making Methods for making an herbal salve, using either the Simpler's Method or the Quick Method. Use this ointment liberally on cuts, scrapes, burns, bites, stings, itchy skin, ringworm, scrofula, eczema, and any injury on which you would normally use an antibiotic salve or cream. *Note:* Do not use it on deep cuts, as comfrey will heal the surface tissues first while the deeper layers of tissue may harbor infectious bacteria. For deep cuts, third-degree burns, and severe injuries, consult a health care practitioner or go to the emergency room.

Yields 2 cups

2 tablespoons yarrow
2 tablespoons comfrey, chopped
2 tablespoons elder leaves, chopped
2 tablespoons red clover blossoms
2 tablespoons plantain leaves, chopped
1 tablespoon peppermint leaves, chopped
1 tablespoon calendula petals
1 teaspoon hemlock tips (and/ or cedar or juniper tips)
15 drops rosemary essential oil
15 drops clove essential oil
2 cups olive and/or canola oil
½ cup beeswax

FAMOUS IN TEXAS

I'm always thankful to hear people's positive responses to my Rosemary's Blessing First Aid Ointment: "This stuff is a miracle!" "I put it on my baby's bottom, and all the rash has gone!" "We are using it up. It's working." The best affirmation for its success was when a husband and wife approached me at my farmer's market booth with an empty Rosemary's Blessing jar. The man scanned my tables, picked up a new jar, and held it high. He was beaming. "Here it is!" he said to his wife. "I found it!" His wife smiled at me. "He won't use anything else. He's been so excited to come back to the island just so he can get more of that stuff." The man stood beside me holding his jar of salve, and his wife took a picture of us. "We're from Texas," he said. "You're famous in Texas."

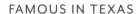

Infection Ointment

Yields 1 cup

2 tablespoons elder leaves, chopped

1 tablespoon dried arnica

1 tablespoon hemlock tips

1 teaspoon powdered goldenseal root

1 teaspoon balm of Gilead buds, crushed

1 cup olive and/or canola oil

¼ cup beeswax

This is a strong ointment for treating infections and stubborn wounds. Similar to the "black salves" of antiquity, it is dark in color and is strongly antibacterial. Keep in mind that both arnica and goldenseal (Hydrastis canadensis) are at risk for overharvesting and are difficult to cultivate. Use common alternatives when possible; barberry root and Oregon grape root make good substitutes for goldenseal.

Follow the instructions in chapter 4: Medicine-Making Methods for making an herbal salve, using either the Simpler's Method or the Quick Method. Use this ointment sparingly.

Quick Yarrow Compress

We're lucky to have such a prominent and easy-to-gather herb as yarrow for a reliable wound healer.

Follow the instructions in chapter 4: Medicine-Making Methods for making a compress or a poultice. Apply for 30 minutes at a time, changing cloths to keep the application hot.

Yields 2 cups

2 large handfuls fresh
    yarrow leaves, chopped
2 cups fresh water
2 cotton or flannel cloths

BEE STINGS

When poison or a foreign object enters the outer tissues of the body (such as through snakebite, nettle stings, bee stings, and even splinters), consider this an opportunity to use so-called black salves, or drawing salves. These special, dark, thick ointments were, long ago, the first recourse for people living in the country, outback, or prairie. Frequently they were "fatted" with goose grease, bear grease, or some other rendered animal fat. We can still use these effective drawing herbs today, substituting pleasant-smelling beeswax for the fat.

Quick Plantain Poultice

Plantain leaves have the uncanny ability to draw objects from the body: splinters, poison, and sometimes even cysts and tumors. For this reason, it was often used as the primary ingredient in old-fashioned drawing salves. I've had great results healing bee stings with this simple and wonderful plant.

1 handful fresh plantain
    leaves

If you've been stung by a bee, pluck a plantain leaf (either large leaf or lance leaf). Briefly macerate it in your mouth for a few seconds, chewing it to obtain a rough but juicy material. Remove it from your mouth and apply it directly to the sting. You'll feel it heat up quickly. Once the heat has dissipated, remove the leaf and prepare another in the same way. You may go through 5 to 15 leaves in this fashion as the leaves pull the venom from the skin. The itch will quickly subside.

Red Clover Bee Sting Cream

Yields approximately ¼ cup

2 to 4 red clover blossoms, shredded

1 large (hand-size) plantain leaf, chopped

4 tablespoons vegetable oil

1 tablespoon beeswax

1 teaspoon baking soda

Soothing red clover cools the heat of an aching bee sting, and plantain and baking soda pull the poison from the skin, making this a fast and effective all-natural bee sting rememdy.

Mix the red clover and plantain in the oil; simmer on low heat for 5 minutes. Strain the oil and pour it back in the pot. Slowly melt the beeswax into the oil, and as it dissolves, stir in the baking soda. As soon as the beeswax melts, pour the mixture into a small glass jar and allow it to cool. Apply the cream directly to stings.

BURNS AND SUNBURN

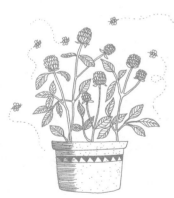

Large or third-degree burns must be treated by a health care practitioner. Sunburn can be surprisingly acute and can range from a mild irritation to a full-blown, third-degree, blistering burn. Fever, nausea, and even vomiting often accompany bad burns. In severe cases, you need to keep hydrated and see a health care practitioner. For small burns or mild to moderate sunburns, begin the healing process by treating the tissues to soothing lavender, marshmallow, and plantain.

Lavender has been hailed as a key burn-healing plant since its "discovery," detailed in the French chemist and perfumer Rene-Maurice Gattefosse's 1937 book Aromatherapie: Les Huiles Essentielles Hormones Vegetales. *The story of his discovery is nearly legendary: while working in his laboratory, Gattefosse burned his hand and, in pain, reached for something to apply to the burn. By chance, he grabbed a recently made batch of pure lavender essential oil. To his surprise, the burn healed quickly without leaving scar tissue.*

The oil in the Lavender-Beeswax Salve nourishes your skin while the beeswax provides a moisture barrier, keeping infection at bay and sealing in your body's healing fluids. Make this balm and keep it in the first aid cabinet for emergencies.

Yields 1 cup

1 cup fresh lavender
  flowers (or ½ cup dried)
1 cup vegetable oil (olive or
  canola)
¼ cup beeswax
8 drops lavender essential
  oil

Follow the instructions in chapter 4: Medicine-Making Methods for making an herbal salve. Apply gently as needed to fresh burns, taking care not to pull the skin. Cover the treated area lightly with a sterile bandage, drink plenty of water, and rest.

Marshmallow-Plantain Burn Remedy ꙮ

For mild burns where the skin is not broken, carefully apply this soothing remedy.

Yields 2 cups

For a Compress

In a wide, shallow pan, bring the water to a simmer. Stir in the herbs, cover, and heat, about 10 minutes. Strain the herbs and compost them. Save the liquid and return it to the pan. Soak a clean cotton or wool cloth in the liquid, gently wring out the excess, and apply the wet cloth directly to the burn.

½ cup dried marshmallow
  root
½ cup dried plantain leaves
  (or 1 cup fresh)
2 cups water

For a Poultice

In a wide, shallow pan, bring the water to a simmer. Stir in the herbs, cover, and heat until they are tender and plump, about 30 minutes. Carefully strain the herbs, lightly squeeze out the excess water, and apply the wet herbs directly to the burn. Hold them in place with a clean cotton gauze or cloth, and reapply every 10 or 15 minutes as the material cools.

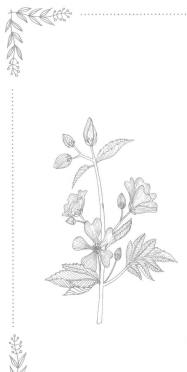

MARSHMALLOW
Althaea officinalis

The lovely mallow has been cultivated widely for garden and ornamental use. The leaves resemble maple leaves, and the flower resembles a geranium blossom; the plant is compact and grows up to three feet high. The edible leaves make a mild medicine, but the fresh root is the most potent. It's mucilaginous—high in soothing properties that make it an excellent remedy for coughs, sore nipples, cracked skin, open sores, ulcers, and digestive complaints. Make a tea, and you'll quickly see the value of this root: it gets thick and slimy. This may not look appetizing, but it certainly is useful as a medicine—consider all the inflamed, hot, swollen, crusty, and hacking ailments that can benefit from a natural soothing gel.

INSECT REPELLENT

You don't need nasty chemical-laden sprays from the store to keep bugs away, especially those that contain DEET, which has been proven carcinogenic. Anything applied to the skin is rapidly absorbed, so use the following all-natural spray on clothing, socks, shoes, and sparingly on the skin. I do not recommend its use on babies.

Bye-Bye Bugs Insect Repellent Spray

Sweet fern is a lovely plant that grows wild here on Martha's Vineyard and along the entire East Coast. Because of its aromatic scent, the Wampanoag and other peoples have long used it as an insect repellent. Combined with sage, this smell-good spray repels flies, mosquitoes, gnats, no-see-ums, and possibly ticks.

In a glass jar with a tight-fitting lid, soak the sweet fern and sage in the witch hazel and water for two weeks. Strain the liquid, and add 20 to 30 drops total of the essential oils of your choice. Store it in spray bottles for easy application. This makes a strong-smelling insect repellent that should be kept away from the eyes and *not* used on infants.

Yields 2 cups

1 cup fresh sweet fern leaves, chopped
1 cup fresh sage, chopped
1 cup witch hazel
1 cup water (preferably distilled)
Essential oils (good bug-repelling oils include citronella, lemongrass, peppermint, camphor, and rosemary)

POISON IVY AND POISON OAK

Poison ivy, in addition to being the name of the plant, is actually our term for an allergic skin reaction received on contact with the plant's stem, leaves, or root. Some people experience rashes and some don't; when they do, the blisters erupt into boils on the skin, and I believe the plant's chemicals actually pass through the bloodstream to various parts of the body. More research should be done on the spreading of this allergic reaction as there is much myth and little science to tell us exactly how this plant poisons us. For best results for stubborn cases, combine the following astringent remedies with the Extra Strength Liver Cleanse in chapter 15, which will support the liver's metabolic function.

Magical Jewelweed-Plantain Cubes

Yields approximately 12 to 15 cubes

3 to 5 fresh jewelweed stalks with leaves
1 large handful fresh plantain leaves

Jewelweed is a wild member of the Impatiens family and is a lovely wildflower in eastern America. Its orange and yellow flowers and silvery leaves grow on a tall, hollow stalk, and inside the stalk is the "juice" that is prized by herbalists for treating poison ivy. You can break the stalk and rub the juice directly on the skin, or prepare the following cubes to preserve the juice for use any time in the summer and fall.

Coarsely chop the stalks and leaves of both plants into chunks, saving as much juice as possible. Place everything in a blender and process . Pour the mixture through a sieve or strainer and press out as much juice as possible. Pour this juice into ice cube trays, label them, and freeze. These magical cubes will be ready when you need them; simply rub a cube on affected skin.

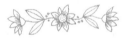

The astringent herbs in this spray are wonderful for drying the annoying blisters associated with poison ivy and poison oak. Preserved with witch hazel, this is a wonderful external formula for drying up the infection and stopping its spread.

Coarsely chop the jewelweed, saving as much juice as possible. Combine all the ingredients in a 1-quart glass jar, and steep in a dark cabinet for two weeks. Strain the mixture and store it in a spray bottle. Apply to the skin as needed.

Yields 2 cups

1 large (3-foot-high)
    jewelweed stalk

¼ cup fresh red clover
    blossoms

¼ cup fresh lady's mantle

¼ cup fresh plantain

¼ cup fresh yarrow

¼ cup fresh sage

1 cup witch hazel

1 cup water

COLD SORES

Herpes lesions are caused by a disturbing and pervasive viral infection. Herpes can inflict wounds on the body in worrisome places, usually the genital area and the lips, and it's spread by simple skin-to-skin contact. To combat this virus and heal the painful lesions, follow these protocols:

· Take acidophilus and other probiotics regularly.
· Try antiviral herbs such as lemon balm, Saint-John's-wort, and
  echinacea as teas, tinctures, and capsules.
· Be sure not to pick at or scratch the lesions. Use soothing emollient
  salves such as the following lemon balm ointment or a calendula or
  plantain salve to reduce the itch and keep the area soothed.

Lemon Balm Cold Sore Ointment

Yields 1 cup

¾ cup packed fresh lemon
balm

¼ cup packed fresh Saint-
John's-wort

¼ cup dried wild yam root
(optional)

1 cup olive or canola oil

¼ cup beeswax, chopped

Clinical studies have shown lemon balm and other mints to be strongly antiviral against both known herpes viruses—the cold sore (HSV-1), and the genital virus (HSV-2). By itself or combined with Saint-John's-wort and wild yam (other antiviral herbs), it is a safe and effective treatment for herpes sores wherever they may appear. In conjunction with this topical treatment, drink the Herpy Tea (the recipe follows) regularly.

Follow the instructions in chapter 4: Medicine-Making Methods for making herbal salves. Apply the ointment frequently to the affected area.

Herpy Tea

Yields 1 quart

1 tablespoon dried wild
yam root

1 tablespoon dried
echinacea root

1 quart boiling water

2 tablespoons dried lemon
balm leaves

2 tablespoons dried Saint-
John's-wort leaves and
flowers

Cold sores must be addressed both externally (for the wound) and internally (for the virus). This tea is a delicious and effective antiviral that provides protection to the body while it addresses the virus.

In a saucepan, combine the wild yam and echinacea roots; cover them with the water. Cover the pan tightly and bring to a boil. Immediately reduce the heat and simmer 30 minutes. Lift the lid and carefully add the lemon balm and Saint-John's-wort. Steep for an additional 5 to 8 minutes. Strain the tea and sweeten as desired. Drink 2 to 3 cups daily.

Chapter Twelve

HAPPY HEART

The heart is the seat of the soul, according to some ancient traditions, and Ayurveda considers the heart the seat of consciousness. "Caring for the heart" can mean literally caring for the muscle, or it can be more ephemeral, referring to our love, our soul, or a grieving process. This chapter addresses remedies for the heart muscle and circulation; for remedies to address emotional concerns, see chapter 16: Mind and Spirit.

Often when people have issues with their heart muscle, they experience certain symptoms: low blood pressure, high blood pressure, poor circulation, or arrhythmia (irregular heartbeat). Since the heart is an incredibly vital organ, it is not within the scope of this book to recommend remedies for serious cardiac problems, but we will touch on a few ways you can address simple cardiac care in tandem with your health care practitioner's advice. As always, and especially with the heart, give your health care practitioner a list (or samples) of the herbs you take, since some of them may be contraindicated with certain prescription medications.

For centuries herbalists have sought natural remedies for the heart muscle. William Withering, of Shropshire, England, was the first to publish his findings about foxglove (the biennial *Digitalis*), though he actually learned about the remedy from Wise Women all over Britain who historically had used it to treat their families. When I visited Shropshire years ago, I naively expected to find an ancient village overgrown with great hedges of foxglove, testament to its rightful place in history. Instead I found a contemporary town and bus station with little evidence of the historic scientific discovery—and even less foxglove. Withering took credit for the women's knowledge, and medical research has since proven the effectiveness of foxglove, ultimately corroborating what those women knew: it has a tremendous effect on the contractility of the heart muscle. Because of its power, only professional herbalists should administer foxglove.

Thankfully, milder herbs are available that perform much the same function, in combination with a good diet of fresh fruits and vegetables, coarse whole grains (not refined), low intake of table salt and salty foods, plenty of fresh water, and moderate weight-bearing exercise. Hawthorn (*Cretaegus oxyacanthoides* and other species) is one of the most beloved cardiac herbs, as its flowers, leaves, and berries can be prepared as a tea, tincture, powdered herb, or even a paste or jam. Widely accepted as a cardiac tonic, hawthorn is used to address cardiovascular disease and heart congestion and to increase coronary and myocardial circulation. It works by dilating the coronary arteries to allow for greater blood flow and improves nutrient uptake by the heart's cells.

Many herbs rightfully take their place in the apothecary's cabinet for the cardiovascular system. Welsh herbalist David Hoffmann notes that even innocent borage, for example, is prized as a cardiac tonic; he says, "Consider the cordial, a warming drink and a word for heartfelt friendliness. The original cordial was a medieval drink based on borage (*Borago officinalis*) that warmed the heart and gave the person *heart*."

HEART TONICS

The herbs in these remedies are traditional heart tonics, meaning they directly nourish and physically affect heart muscle contractility, strength, and resilience. These herbs, in various combinations, have been used for centuries and have the added benefit of giving you energy and a sense of vitality.

Heart-Warming Tea

This gentle heart tonic is safe to take long term as a remedy for high blood pressure and heart palpitations.

Combine the herbs in a 1-quart glass jar, cover with enough boiling water to fill the jar. Steep for 15 to 20 minutes, strain the tea, and drink it throughout the day.

Yields 1 quart

2 tablespoons dried
    hawthorn flowers,
    leaves, and/or berries
2 tablespoons dried borage
    leaves and/or flowers

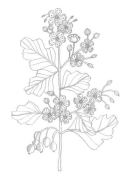

Heart-Strengthening Tonic

This is a nerve-soothing tea to strengthen the muscle action of the heart. It can be very warming and is good in situations where the heart (and/or emotions) feels stagnant, cold, or "stuck."

Yields 1 quart

Combine the first three herbs in a 1-quart glass jar. Pour enough boiling water over them to fill the jar. Steep for 8 minutes. Add the motherwort and yarrow, and steep for an additional 2 to 3 minutes but no longer, as these herbs are quite bitter. Strain the liquid, and sweeten to taste. Drink it freely.

2 tablespoons dried
    hawthorn flowers,
    leaves, and/or berries
2 tablespoons dried
    peppermint
1 tablespoon dried ginkgo
    leaves
1 teaspoon dried
    motherwort herb
¼ teaspoon dried yarrow
    leaves
Honey, stevia, or maple
    syrup, to taste

❧ Hearty Berry Jam

Yields approximately 2 pints   *Enjoy this nourishing spread on bread and bagels.*

1 cup blueberries

1 cup bilberries

1 cup hawthorn berries

2 cups sugar

2 tablespoons lemon juice

In a large pot, mash the berries and sugar together. Bring them to a boil over high heat and immediately reduce the heat to a simmer. Simmer for 20 minutes, removing any scum or foam from the top and stirring frequently. Stir in the lemon juice. Pour the mixture into 1-pint glass canning jars with lids. Store them in the refrigerator for immediate consumption; to preserve for future use, process them in a water bath for 20 minutes or in a pressure cooker according to the manufacturer's directions.

CIRCULATION

Some herbs are especially adept at improving the circulatory system and increasing both the quality and strength of blood flow. Combined with movement and proper exercise, they are a valuable treatment for cold extremities, weak heart function, and poor circulation.

❧ Cold Hands/Cold Feet Circulatory Tea

Yields 1 quart

2 tablespoons dried prickly ash bark

2 tablespoons dried ginkgo leaves

2 teaspoons dried yarrow

1 quart boiling water

Drink this bitter, hot tea to relieve cold extremities, varicose veins, chilblains, leg cramps, and arthritic stiffness. Prickly ash (Zanthoxylum americanum) is renowned for getting blood to flow freely.

Combine the herbs in a 1-quart glass jar, and cover them with the water. Steep for 8 to 10 minutes. Strain the tea and sweeten as desired. Drink it throughout the day.

Circulation Celebration Cocoa

This is a delicious, heart-warming, circulation-stimulating brew.

Combine the herbs in a soup pot and pour the water over them. Steep for 8 to 10 minutes; strain the liquid and return it to the pot. Whisk in the cocoa, sugar, and milk. Steep for another 5 minutes, stirring frequently. Serve this drink hot. To make it festive, serve it with a peppermint stick. Refrigerate any leftover cocoa and use within 24 hours.

Yields 1 quart

2 teaspoons dried prickly ash bark

2 teaspoons dried peppermint leaves

1 teaspoon dried yarrow herb

1 quart boiling water

4 teaspoons cocoa powder

2 teaspoons sugar

½ cup milk

Tangy Circulation Drink

This is a citrusy hot drink to improve blood flow and care for the heart.

Combine all the herbs except the cayenne pepper in a 1-quart glass jar, and cover them with enough boiling water to fill the jar. Steep for 8 to 12 minutes, then strain the liquid. Stir in the dash of cayenne (or as much as you can stand), lemon juice, and maple syrup. Drink it freely; it's wonderful on a cold winter day! Refrigerate any leftover beverage and use within 24 hours.

Yields 1 quart

2 tablespoons dried lemon balm

2 tablespoons dried lemongrass

2 tablespoons dried ginkgo

¼ teaspoon dried ginger (granules or powder)

Dash cayenne pepper

2 teaspoons lemon juice

1 teaspoon maple syrup

Warming Hand and Foot Salve

Yields 1 cup

1 cup fresh peppermint, chopped

½ cup fresh ginger, chopped (including skin)

1 cup olive or canola oil

¼ cup beeswax

This topical salve made with warming herbs brings blood flow to the area where it is applied. It's nice to put this salve on chilly feet at night—and cover them with cotton socks if desired.

Follow the instructions in chapter 4: Medicine-Making Methods for making an herbal salve. Apply it liberally to hands or feet, and be sure to keep it out of the eyes.

DIURETICS AND BITTERS

Bitter herbs stimulate digestion and act as nourishing diuretics to ease the pressure on the entire circulatory system. For more recipes with bitters, see chapter 13: Tummy Health.

Hearty Bitters

Yields 2 cups

1 teaspoon dried motherwort leaves, chopped (or 3 teaspoons fresh)

1 teaspoon dried dandelion leaves, chopped (or 3 teaspoons fresh)

2 cups boiling water

Honey, molasses, or maple syrup

This recipe is especially helpful for conditions of cardiac stress due to anxiety. Motherwort and dandelion are both diuretic, relieving the pressure on heart function, and their bitter taste stimulates digestive function, which is particularly useful when anxious tension causes indigestion or heartburn.

Chop the herbs, place them in a 1-pint glass jar or teapot, and steep them in the water for 5 to 8 minutes. The longer they brew, the more bitter they will become. Strain the liquid, and sweeten to taste (molasses decreases the bitterness). Take ¼ teaspoon, hot or cold, preferably before meals. Refrigerate the unused portion and use within 2 weeks.

Chapter Thirteen

TUMMY HEALTH

Nothing makes me lose my vitality and luster more quickly than being nauseous. If my stomach hurts or I feel crampy, dizzy, or sick, I can't get work done. Most of us feel this way; nausea impedes our daily life and saps us of our confidence and zest. (If you have sudden, bending-over-double pain, please seek medical attention immediately!) There are many causes of nausea. There are many healing herbal treatments for chronic or mild queasiness, especially when the cause is digestive.

In centuries past, it was the doctor's great joy to "see" the results of a treatment. Practitioners assumed that if the body evacuated liquid, the patient must be getting better. Sick people were given harsh herbs and mineral substances that made them salivate, drool, vomit, expel diarrhea, urinate, cry, and sweat profusely. The poor patients often suffered extreme pain, confusion, and dehydration before they either died or (through no credit to the doctor) lived. Thankfully, we—especially herbalists—now use gentler methods. (For more information on this surprising history, read Barbara Griggs's *Green Pharmacy*.)

Use the following formulas to address cramps, nausea, indigestion, heartburn, ulcers, gas, and bloating. You'll also find formulas and dietary suggestions for relieving constipation and diarrhea.

INDIGESTION

The best methods for treating nausea and digestive complaints involve aromatic (often culinary) herbs that soothe the stomach lining and ease pain in the digestive tract. Stomach herbs stimulate good digestion and act in many ways: some soothe inflamed tissues; some stimulate gastric and pancreatic juices; some ease constipation; and some relax muscle cramping. As indigestion often causes many of these symptoms, aromatic herbs are among the first to try.

Digestive Aid/Gas Relief Tincture

Yields 2 to 3 cups

2 tablespoons fresh catnip

2 tablespoons fresh dill

2 tablespoons dried chamomile

2 tablespoons dried peppermint

1 teaspoon dried lemon balm

1 teaspoon dried fennel seeds

1 teaspoon dried dandelion leaves

½-inch piece fresh ginger (skin included)

½ teaspoon dried crampbark

2 cups vodka

1 cup water

This has been my best-selling tincture for years. Once, when I was selling at the Merle Watson Festival (MerleFest) outside Boone, North Carolina, a man marched headlong toward my booth. He pushed past other people and made a beeline to my table. Without a word, he searched the display and picked up a Digestive Aid tincture bottle. With an outstretched hand and a loud voice—and a broad smile—he announced to everyone gathered there, "This stuff works!"

The aromatic and fragrant herbs in this formula have been prized since ancient times for healing upset tummies. They are so beloved, in fact, that they are often grown outside the kitchen door and used by people worldwide. Dill, fennel, peppermint, catnip, chamomile, lemon balm—we take them for granted, but they are a godsend when our lives are put on hold because of nausea, gas, and discomfort. Use this formula with confidence when you or a friend or family member suffers digestive-related symptoms such as distended belly, cramps, gas, heartburn, and constipation.

Follow the instructions in chapter 4: Medicine-Making Methods for making an alcohol tincture. Use it as needed when symptoms of indigestion occur. Place 20 to 30 drops in a small amount of cool or warm water, and take it every hour until the indigestion subsides.

If your indigestion is chronic, add the herbs themselves to your daily diet. Often oily, greasy, or acidic foods trigger pain, so avoid these foods.

Cramps Formula

These herbs reduce spasms in the gut, which helps to relieve indigestion and general abdominal cramping.

Follow the instructions in chapter 4: Medicine-Making Methods for making an alcohol tincture, using a 1-pint glass jar instead of the 1-quart jar. Take the tincture in a small amount of water or tea as needed.

Yields 1 cup

1 tablespoon dried wild yam root
1 tablespoon dried crampbark
½ teaspoon dried dill
½ teaspoon dried fennel seeds
½ teaspoon dried catnip
½ cup vodka
½ cup water

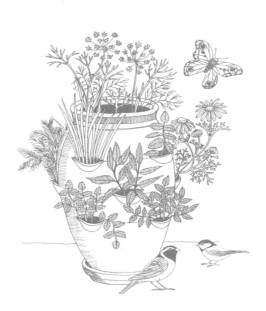

Bitters Tincture

Yields 2 cups

1 teaspoon dried dandelion
   leaves

1 teaspoon dried
   motherwort leaves

1 teaspoon dried raspberry
   leaves

1 teaspoon dried yarrow
   leaves

1 teaspoon dried calendula

1 teaspoon dried licorice
   (optional)

1 cup brandy

1 cup water

Bitters, believe it or not, are our friends. They stimulate proper digestion and work hand in hand, so to speak, with the liver. Too bad for us that we eat so many sweets; bitterness is a taste we have largely outgrown—to our detriment.

The bitter tinctures you'll find in the health food store are often made with roots from plants that are endangered or at risk, such as goldenseal. This formula, by contrast, contains herbs and roots that meet my requirements for Essential Herbs based on safety, ease in finding and harvesting, and nonthreatened status. Triple the quantity of herbs if you're using fresh ones.

Follow the instructions in chapter 4: Medicine-Making Methods for making an alcohol tincture, using a 1-pint glass jar instead of the 1-quart jar. Add the licorice if you're using it for children.

Take small doses of this tincture (2 to 5 drops) when experiencing heartburn, indigestion, or problems with bowel movements. Drop it into water or tea, or better yet, right on your tongue.

Menemsha Mint Tea

Yields 1 quart

2 tablespoons dried
   peppermint

2 tablespoons dried
   spearmint

2 tablespoons dried
   hibiscus

1 tablespoon dried
   chamomile (optional)

1 quart boiling water

This tea is useful for hot, sweaty conditions—as when you eat a huge meal and suddenly feel feverish and sluggish. Mint can be cooling, soothing, and refreshing, as well as warming and stimulating. It promotes the production of bile and other digestive "juices" from the pancreas, liver, and gall bladder. The optional chamomile is a nervine, which means it soothes stressed nerves. It's also a mild antispasmodic.

Place the herbs in a teapot and pour the water over them. Steep for 5 to 8 minutes, covered. Strain the tea, and sweeten it lightly as desired. Drink it hot, as needed. Refrigerate any leftover tea and use within 24 hours.

ULCERS AND HEARTBURN

Demulcent herbs are those high in mucilage, a gummy or stringy substance that makes them ideal for soothing the gastrointestinal tract. Mucilaginous plants, including plantain and marshmallow, are ideal in teas or capsules to ease pain and reduce inflammation that can lead to heartburn or the development of ulcers. Licorice is approved by Commission E, the German counterpart of the U.S. Food and Drug Administration, as a remedy for ulcers.

Heartburn Tea

Drink this soothing tea when the pain of heartburn causes a sharp intake of breath; achiness; and the classic burning sensation associated with over-eating, eating fried foods, and eating while stressed. The infusion is slightly thicker than regular teas, and it doesn't keep well, so drink it immediately.

Place the herbs in a teapot with the water and steep for 8 to 10 minutes. The water will turn a thick, dark green and, depending on your perspective, will look either slimy or soothing. Strain the tea, and sweeten with honey to taste. Drink ½ cup, warm, every 30 minutes until symptoms subside. (See also see the Lemon Balm Tincture later in this section.)

Yields 1 cup

1 tablespoon fresh plantain
   leaves, chopped
2 tablespoons fresh
   plantain seeds, stripped
   from the seed stalk
1 teaspoon licorice root
1 cup water
Honey

Ulcer Marshmallow Tea

Yields 1 cup

1 teaspoon dried
    marshmallow root,
    chopped

1 teaspoon dried licorice
    root, chopped

1 teaspoon dried lemon
    balm leaves, chopped

1 cup boiling water

Ulcers can be caused by bacteria and by the body's poor immune function following stress. This tea will soothe the intestinal lining; some herbalists use marshmallow as an immune stimulant, and the roots may contain infection-fighting properties that make it ideal for gastrointestinal infections.

Combine the herbs in an enamel or glass pot and pour the water over them. Steep for 5 to 8 minutes. Strain the tea. Drink a cup warm every hour for up to 4 hours for acute ulcer pain, or drink a cup 3 to 4 times daily. The infusion is slightly thicker than regular teas and it doesn't keep well, so drink it immediately.

Aquinnah Cliffs Licorice Tea

Yields 1 quart

2 tablespoons dried
    licorice root

1 1-inch cinnamon stick

1 tablespoon dried orange
    peel (or 3 tablespoons
    fresh)

1 tablespoon dried nettle
    leaves

1 tablespoon cardamom
    pods

1 teaspoon anise seeds

2 to 3 whole cloves

This regally smooth brew is a favorite on Martha's Vineyard, where the winters are long, cold, and quiet. Licorice is a prime cough remedy and wonderfully useful for digestive complaints. Brew a hot cup of this tea when your tummy is feeling out of sorts; my children love it and ask for it regularly. The orange peel can be fresh or dried.

Combine all the ingredients in a 1-quart glass jar. Pour enough water over them to fill the jar. Steep for 10 to 15 minutes. Strain the tea (no sweetener is necessary) and keep it in a thermos so you can enjoy hot cups throughout the day.

Lemon Balm Tincture

Melissa officinalis, or lemon balm, is one of nature's most wonderful herbs, especially as a nervine or "nerve tonic." I recommend planting this herb above all others, whether you have a large garden or only a pot on the porch. Lemony, fragrant, tasty, and infinitely useful, this herb is prized for internal and external remedies the world over. Lemon balm tames jangled nerves, allowing the body to adjust to stresses that may otherwise prove overwhelming. Use it whenever you're feeling anxious, unable to concentrate, or scattered in many directions at once.

Follow the instructions in chapter 4: Medicine-Making Methods for making an alcohol tincture. Use the dosage guidelines on pages 287–90.

Yields 2 cups

2 cups fresh lemon balm, chopped (or 1 cup dried)
1 cup grain alcohol (such as vodka or brandy)
½ cup vegetable glycerin
½ cup water

Lemon Balm Tea

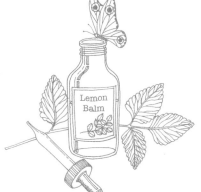

This tea is great for soothing upset nerves and tummies.

Place the lemon balm in a 1-quart glass jar. Pour enough boiling water over it to fill the jar. Steep for 10 to 12 minutes or overnight, tightly covered. Strain the tea and store it in a thermos. Drink it freely.

Yields 1 quart

1 cup dried lemon balm (or 3 cups fresh)

CONSTIPATION

Sluggish or slow bowel movements are not only irritating, they can be the sign of other problems that will increase if not addressed. Constipation means the body is unable to remove waste products efficiently, so other organs of elimination (such as the kidneys, liver, and skin) become stressed or overworked. There are several ways to keep regular movements:

- Use the following Loosening Formula and drink more than enough fresh, clean water.
- Be sure to eat fiber-rich, nonrefined foods such as wheat bran, whole grains, and dried fruits (especially dates, figs, prunes, and raisins).
- Eat mucilaginous foods such as plantain seeds (which are wonderful sprinkled on oatmeal).
- Avoid dairy products such as cheese and milk.
- Increase the amount of yogurt in your diet, and take acidophilus (liquid or tablets).

Loosening Formula

Yields 1½ cups

1 teaspoon dried marshmallow root, chopped

½ teaspoon dried licorice root

½ teaspoon dried plantain seeds

½ teaspoon dried nettle leaves

⅛ teaspoon dried dill

These herbs provide bulk and can be eaten as foods, though this recipe for a tea offers many of the same benefits—including extra water for hydration. The lightly laxative herbs stimulate proper movement without being as strong as a purgative such as senna.

Combine all the ingredients in a 1-pint glass jar. Pour enough boiling water over them to fill the jar. Steep for 10 to 12 minutes, then strain the tea into a thermos. Sip ½ cup every 20 minutes.

DIARRHEA

Everyone occasionally suffers from this annoying and painful symptom of indigestion. It frequently presents itself during colds and flu as the body attempts to purge itself of bacterial and viral infections, so don't be afraid to use this tea when you have a cold. In fact, yarrow is a wonderful influenza herb, and sage can dry up excess mucous production in the sinuses. It is another example of how herbs work synergistically to help us meet our health needs.

For diarrhea, powdered herbs can be wonderfully beneficial. They are simply dried herbs that have been pulverized and sifted to a fine consistency.

When using powders, try to dry and grind your own herbs (using a coffee grinder dedicated to herbs), straining them through a sifter first and then through one or two layers of cheesecloth for an extrafine texture. If you purchase powdered herbs, look for those with bold, rich colors and scents. Old and stale powders will be dull and lifeless. There are many ways to use powders: put them in capsules; sprinkle them in warm honey to spread on toast; sprinkle them on oatmeal, grits, or a cream of wheat cereal; blend them into salad dressings; or mix them in grapefruit or orange juice.

Adult Healing Tea

This is a lip-puckering, astringent brew that will help the body tighten and hold in liquid while, at the same time, reducing spasms in the intestinal tract. It is best for adults. For children, see the recipe for Children's Raspberry Formula with Yarrow in chapter 6: For Infant and Child.

Combine the herbs in a glass, enamel, or porcelain teapot, and pour the water over them. Steep for 5 to 8 minutes, then strain the tea and sweeten as desired. Drink ½ to 1 cup every 30 minutes. Be sure to drink plenty of water in between.

Yields 2 cups

1 teaspoon dried sage leaves
½ teaspoon dried yarrow leaves
½ teaspoon dried raspberry leaves
¼ teaspoon crampbark
2 cups boiling fresh water

Pick-Me-Up Powder for Diarrhea

Yields 1 cup

1/3 cup powdered sage

1/3 cup powdered
    raspberry leaves

1/3 cup powdered
    marshmallow root

This remedy also uses astringent herbs combined with demulcent, or soothing, ones to relieve the cramps and water loss of diarrhea. Put the powder in capsules, or mix it with honey or juice.

Combine all the powders thoroughly in a glass bowl. If you like, put them in gelatin capsules and take 6 to 12 capsules daily. Otherwise, store the powder mixture in a small jar with a tight-fitting lid. Take 1 teaspoon 3 times daily by stirring the powder into juice or other foods.

Recovery Powdered Honey

Yields 2 cups

1 tablespoon powdered
    slippery elm

1 tablespoon powdered
    echinacea

1 teaspoon powdered
    marshmallow root

2 cups honey

*Slippery elm powder (*Ulmus rubra, *formerly* Ulmus fulva) *from the inner bark of the elm) has long been loved by herbalists as a mild, nourishing, and soothing way to restore vitality and balance to the body after an illness. Combined with infection-fighting echinacea, soothing marshmallow root, and mineral-rich honey, it eases the body back into health after a bout of diarrhea or other abdominal illness.*

Combine the powders in a stainless steel pot and place on the stove. Pour the honey over them, and gently heat the mixture only enough to melt the honey to a liquid consistency. As soon as the herbs can easily be stirred through the honey, remove the pot from the heat and pour the honey into a glass jar with a tight-fitting lid. Cap the jar and let it cool.

There are many ways to use this nourishing remedy: taken by the spoonful or several teaspoons daily, either drizzled over oatmeal, stirred into tea, or spread on toast.

Chapter Fourteen

ACHES AND PAINS

Our bodies constantly bend, lift, turn, and reach. Or as medical terminology puts it, we flex, extend, and rotate. Our joints allow us to be graceful and effective at what we wish to accomplish. We are naturally supple, resilient, and mobile, but if our joints ache or have become stiff or painful, we quickly realize how important a healthy, balanced body is. Many common botanicals, applied topically or taken internally, act as anti-inflammatories and analgesics (herbs that reduce inflammation and ease pain).

HEADACHE

There are two primary types of headaches: tension and vascular (or migraine). The former is often caused by stress or emotional irritation. The tension causes you to constrict your neck and shoulder muscles and generally tighten your body, which results in pain in the head, neck, shoulders, and eyes. Vascular headaches appears to be related to involuntary constriction of the blood vessels in the brain. Migraines can be caused by a variety of (primarily) internal triggers: the body's allergic reaction to foods, spinal damage that needs correction, or hormonal imbalance. I would also add to this list the headache triggers of illness (influenza or other debilitating viral infections), constipation, liver obstruction, Lyme disease, and the aftereffects of cleanses or certain weight-loss diets.

Discover the cause of your headache. Often this is easy (maybe you fought with someone or participated in an irritating meeting), but sometimes it's not. Did you eat something that disagreed with you? Explore your diet and check for other symptoms throughout your body. Have you been bitten by a tick? Where I live on Martha's Vineyard, headaches and muscle aches are red flags to look for the typical red bull's-eye of an infected tick bite. What about your normal routine? Are you trying out a new diet or have you begun taking a new medication?

Finally, don't ignore headaches reported by children. Though they may be pleas for attention, chronic headaches in children may indicate an emergency condition, such as a brain tumor, and should be addressed.

For an occasional tension headache, try the following.

- Go to sleep. The body can heal itself if given the time.
- Take a warm bath. Tie lavender, passionflower, lemon balm, rose petals, or chamomile in a muslin bag and hold it under the faucet to sent the bathwater.
- Eat something sweet with something sour. Rosemary Gladstar recommends a combination such as applesauce with lemon juice to balance the acid-alkaline ratio in the body.
- Rub your shoulders and loosen your neck muscles with simple head-roll exercises. Stretch your arms out to the side, swing your body to loosen all the muscles, and go for a walk in the fresh air.
- Gently rub Lavender Massage Oil (recipe in this section) on your temples and wrists.

The root of valerian is used as a relatively strong sedative. Taken as a hot tea, along with soothing chamomile and regenerative red clover, this herb brings sleep so that all the body's systems can begin healing.

In a 1-quart glass jar, combine the herbs and pour enough boiling water over them to fill the jar. Steep for 5 to 8 minutes, strain the tea, and sweeten if desired. Sip ½ cup every 15 minutes for 45 minutes before going to bed.

Yields 1 quart

2 tablespoons dried chamomile
1 tablespoon dried valerian root
1 tablespoon dried red clover
1 teaspoon dried lavender
Honey, stevia, or maple syrup, to taste

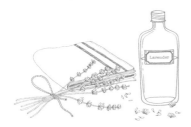

Lavender Compress

Placing a warm, heavenly scented compress on the forehead or temples will often signal to the brain that it can relax. Lavender is soothing and at the same time uplifting; it can safely be used for any age, at any time, to ease discomfort.

Follow the instructions in chapter 4: Medicine-Making Methods for making a compress. Place the compress on your forehead, lie back, and let the heat penetrate. Keep warm under a blanket, and take this time to clear your mind and rub your neck and shoulders.

Yields 2 cups

1 tablespoon fresh lavender flowers (or 1 teaspoon dried)
1 tablepoon fresh rose petals (or 1 teaspoon dried)
2 cups water

Soothing Skullcap Tea

Yields 1 quart

2 tablespoons dried
    skullcap herb
2 tablespoons dried
    passionflower herb
2 tablespoons dried lemon
    balm
Honey, stevia, or maple
    syrup, to taste

Tiny and diminutive, the skullcap herb (Scutellaria lateriflora from the mint family) is considered a safe and effective nervine tonic; it soothes stressed nerves and helps the body relax "from the mind outward." It's blended here with passionflower (Passiflora incarnata, a sedative) and lemon balm (a rejuvenator) for a combination that is at once calming and healing.

Combine the herbs in a 1-quart glass jar. Pour enough boiling water over them to fill the jar. Steep for 10 to 12 minutes, strain the tea, and sweeten if desired. Sip ½ cup every 30 minutes. Refrigerate any unused portion and use within 24 hours.

Lavender Massage Oil

Yields ½ cup

½ cup dried lavender flowers
½ cup oil (such as
    sunflower, sweet
    almond, safflower, or
    jojoba)

This massage oil is soothing and fragrant.

Follow the instructions in chapter 4: Medicine-Making Methods for making an herbal oil. Pour a small amount of this lovely, soothing oil onto your fingers or into the palm of your hand and apply it to your temples, neck, wrists, and shoulders with slow, circular motions. Breathe deeply, and leave it on all day and night. Store the final product in a cool, dark cabinet.

Head-Cramp Formula

Turmeric is used as an anti-inflammatory for various parts of the body, including the digestive tract and the muscular system. Combined with feverfew, which has an "affinity" for the head, its anti-inflammatory actions are guided to exactly where they are needed: the head. Use this tincture for tension and vascular headaches along with the previously mentioned remedies.

Follow in chapter 4: Medicine-Making Methods the instructions for making an alcohol tincture, using a 1-pint glass jar instead of the 1-quart jar. Take ½ to 1 teaspoon in a small amount of water, tea, or juice 3 times daily as needed. Drink plenty of water to keep hydrated.

Yields 2 cups

1 tablespoon powdered
  turmeric
1 tablespoon dried
  crampbark
1 tablespoon dried
  feverfew herb
1 cup vodka
½ cup glycerin
½ cup water

Body Ache Remedy

This is a bitter yet effective remedy for headaches associated with colds, flu, and other illnesses.

Follow the instructions in chapter 4: Medicine-Making Methods for making an herbal infusion. Take ½ cup every hour as needed.

Yields 2 cups

2 teaspoons dried red
  clover
1 teaspoon dried boneset
1 teaspoon dried
  crampbark
1 teaspoon dried
  chamomile

MUSCLE AND JOINT PAIN

Many of our Essential Herbs—such as ginger, yarrow, lavender, lemon balm, peppermint, and nettle—ease aches, arthritis, rheumatism, gout, and joint pain. Nettle has historically been used topically to "burn" or "sting" the ache out of muscles; it was considered rubefacient because the formic acid in its hairs would sting the skin and cause it to redden like a ruby. This was a painful (if effective) remedy. The remedies in this section are more appealing and comfortable and equally effective. Still, I can't overstate how important warmth and heat are to easing the distress of sore, stiff muscles and joints; thus, most of the following remedies employ warmth and moisture.

The body's joints allow it to move in anatomically amazing directions. The bones are connected with tendons, ligaments, and cartilage that, when injured, react with swelling, inflammation, and pain.

When an injury occurs, apply first aid as well as ice or heat, lift the appendage above your head to drain fluids and reduce swelling, and wear a brace as appropriate. The following all-natural remedies will ease congestion of the joint and hasten healing.

Muscle Ache Oil

Yields 1 cup

½ cup fresh yarrow leaves, lightly wilted and chopped
½ cup fresh peppermint leaves (not spearmint), lightly wilted and chopped
1 cup vegetable oil

Yarrow and peppermint are both stimulating, especially when rubbed into the skin as an oil application.

Combine the herbs in a glass or enamel pot and pour the oil over them. Stirring frequently, heat the mixture very gently on low for 10 to 15 minutes. Strain the oil, pour it into a clean bottle, and label it. Warm it again before applying it to the skin; allow it to stay on the skin as long as possible before washing. For best results, rub the oil in and cover the area with a cloth and a hot water bottle.

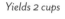

A compress (also called a fomentation) is simply a cotton, wool, or flannel cloth that has been soaked in a medicinal tea and is applied warm to the skin.

Follow the instructions in chapter 4: Medicine-Making Methods for making a compress. Keep reapplying compresses for an hour or as long as the tea remains hot.

Yields 2 cups

½ cup fresh ginger, chopped (skin included)

½ cup fresh peppermint or yarrow leaves, chopped

½ cup fresh Saint-John's-wort leaves and flowers, chopped

½ cup fresh mullein flowers

2 cups boiling water

Mustard Plaster for Sprains

A variation on the typical poultice, this warming, deeply penetrating plaster is made with powdered mustard seed. Be gentle to sensitive skin and leave it on only as long as it is tolerable. This recipe is adapted from the herbalist James Green's The Herbal Medicine-Maker's Handbook.

In a bowl, blend the mustard powder with ½ cup warm water; set aside. In another bowl, blend the flaxseed with the remaining ½ cup warm water. Mix the pastes together to form a thick but spreadable paste (add warm water 1 teaspoon at a time, if necessary, to achieve the right consistency).

Cover or wrap the affected joint with a piece of thin fabric to protect the skin and keep the plaster from sticking. With your fingers, apply the paste thickly over the fabric, all around the joint.

Yields 1 cup

½ cup powdered mustard seed (not squirtable kitchen mustard)

1 teaspoon powdered ginger

1 cup warm water, divided

1 cup ground flaxseed

Cover the paste with a thicker cloth and apply a hot water bottle if desired. Rest, preferably with the affected joint at head-height. Leave the plaster in place for 8 to 10 minutes and promptly wipe off, cleaning the area with warm, soapy water with a pinch of baking soda mixed in.

Arnica Liniment

Yields 2 cups

1 cup dried arnica

2 cups vegetable oil (such as sweet almond, grapeseed, or hemp seed)

½ cup beeswax

Essential oils of ginger, clove, rosemary, sweet birch, Scotch pine, and/or wintergreen (a total of 20 drops, only 2 to 3 of which can be wintergreen)

This recipe can be prepared as a rubbing alcohol liniment, but I prefer it as a beeswax salve. Either way, arnica (Arnica montana) is a powerful anti-inflammatory. It's so powerful and effective, in fact, it has been overharvested in the wild, and because it is difficult to cultivate, it is now on the United Plant Savers' To-Watch list. Be mindful of using this plant and don't waste it. The other herbs and essential oils in this formula stimulate blood flow to the painful area for an overall effect of warmth and vigor; this remedy is helpful in cases of injury, rheumatism, arthritis, gout, and sore joints. (Caution: Do not take arnica internally except in homeopathic form.)

Follow the instructions in chapter 4: Medicine-Making Methods on making an herbal salve. Apply the final product liberally to the affected area, being careful to avoid the eyes and sensitive or broken skin. Cover the area with a hot water bottle if desired, and take the Pain Re-Leaf Formula (which follows) as well.

Pain Re-Leaf Formula

This is an effective analgesic against mild pain, slight headaches, and low-grade chronic pain. Used at the first sign of discomfort, this formula will often eliminate the pain before it grows worse.

As a Tincture

Follow the directions in chapter 4: Medicine-Making Methods for making an alcohol tincture, using a 1-pint glass jar instead of a 1-quart jar. Use the dosage guidelines on pages 287–90 and place dose in a small amount of water, juice, or tea.

Yields 2 cups

2 tablespoons fresh meadowsweet

2 tablespoons fresh lavender

2 tablespoons fresh lemon balm

1 tablespoon fresh Saint-John's-wort

1 tablespoon fresh mullein flowers

½ cup vodka or brandy

½ cup vegetable glycerin

¾ cup water

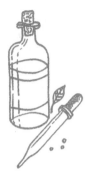

As a Tea

Combine the herbs in a 1-quart glass jar. Pour enough boiling water over them to fill the jar. Steep for 8 to 10 minutes. Strain the tea, sweeten if desired, and drink 1 cup of warm tea every hour until the pain has subsided.

Yields 1 quart

2 tablespoons dried meadowsweet

1 tablespoon dried lavender

1 tablespoon dried lemon balm

1 teaspoon dried Saint-John's-wort

1 teaspoon dried mullein flowers

Honey, stevia, or maple syrup, to taste

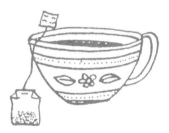

Poppy Pain-Relief Poultice

Yields 2 cups

1 cup poppy seeds

1 large handful dandelion
leaves, chopped

2 cups hot water

The mystical poppy plant (Papaver somniferum) has an ancient history owing to its use as a narcotic when taken internally. The tincture of poppy, or laudanum, used to be, along with calomel, one of the two most frequently prescribed drugs in England, according to renowned herbal historian Barbara Griggs. She lists it as a "splendid painkiller" that was not fully appreciated as a harmful addictive substance that subsequently eroded lives as well as pain. But this is only true when laudanum is taken internally; as an external application, a compress or poultice made with common kitchen poppy seeds is a mild analgesic with no danger of addiction. Dandelion leaf is also considered a mild analgesic.

Place the seeds and leaves in a shallow pan and cover them with the water. Steep 20 to 30 minutes over low heat. Gently strain the herbs and reserve the liquid in the pan. Carefully wrap the herbs in a thin gauze to make a flat "sheet" filled with the herbs, as if you were making a flat pillow. Lay this warm, wet, herb-filled pillow on the painful joint or muscle, cover it with a hot water bottle, and wrap a towel around the whole application. Leave this on the painful joint or muscle for 20 to 30 minutes, or until the application cools. Repeat if necessary. Alternatively, make a compress instead of a poultice by straining the herbs from the pan and soaking a cloth in the hot liquid. Apply this cloth to the affected area, cover with the hot water bottle and towel, and leave on for 20 to 30 minutes, as above.

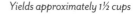
Use this preparation to reduce pain and inflammation associated with sprains; arthritis; rheumatic complaints; and other problems in joints, tendons, and muscles. The fact that these herbs also cleanse and strengthen the liver is key. As a potent diuretic, dandelion rids the liver of allergens that cause inflammation. Note: Because it is a strong diuretic, I recommend using this formula on a one-week-on/one-week-off rotation.

Combine the herbs and roots in a 1-pint glass jar and cover them with the liquids. Follow the instructions in chapter 4: Medicine-Making Methods for making an alcohol tincture. Use the dosage guidelines on pages 287–90.

Yields approximately 1½ cups

½ cup fresh dandelion root, chopped

¼ cup fresh dandelion leaves, chopped

¼ cup fresh meadowsweet (or 2 tablespoons dried)

¼ cup fresh parsley, chopped

1 tablespoon dried turmeric

1 cup grain alcohol (such as vodka or brandy)

¼ cup vegetable glycerin

¼ cup water

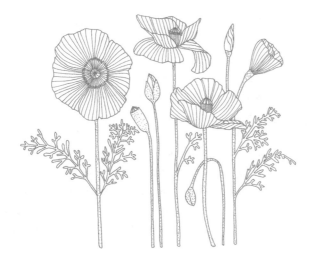

Chapter Fifteen

CLEANSING AND DETOX

Cultures throughout history have found it valuable to "cleanse" and detoxify the body, especially after a long cold winter, an illness such as influenza, or a meal of particularly fatty or heavy foods.

The formulas in this chapter can be rejuvenating and stimulating, allowing the body's many organs of elimination to sweat or otherwise dispel various toxins, such as heavy metals, pollutants, excess minerals, and fats, that can build up in tissue. After a cleanse, people generally feel more alive, "lighter," and more alert.

It's important during any cleanse to make sure you drink an adequate amount of fresh water, usually much more than the recommended eight daily glasses. When detoxifying with bath salts, for example, it is essential to drink water during the bath.

My friend Laurisa shares stories of marvelous cleansing baths taken when she lived in Bora Bora, using some of the thousands of fresh papayas that grew outside her door. She applied the pulp to her skin and sometimes collected volcanic mud for the same purpose. Even today, years later, her skin glows, and I like to think that in addition to her lovely spirit, some of that beauty harkens back to her "spa" days in the tropics.

LIVER

There's a reason *liver* has the word *live* in it. It's one of the key organs for health in the body, contributing to toxic and metabolic waste removal, new red blood cell production, and even spent-hormone removal. The liver also converts ammonia to the less-toxic urea and sends it to the kidneys. Effects of a sick liver include crabbiness, lethargy, weakness, pallor, and even the emotional swings of hormonal imbalance (see chapter 7: Especially for Women for more details on these imbalances). Maintaining the liver is a top priority during any illness and not just as part of "routine" cleansing.

How can you best maintain liver function? For starters, eat as little deep-fried fat as possible. Trans fatty acids and hydrogenated oils require a great effort by the liver to metabolize and export them from the body. Old rancid foods toxify the liver and pollute the bloodstream. Keep sugar intake to a minimum. And consume only the amount of protein required by your level of physical activity; excess protein leads to excess ammonia and more work for the liver.

Certain herbs are hepatics, meaning they act as liver tonics. The roots of dandelion, burdock, and yellow dock and the seeds of milk thistle contain phytochemicals that stimulate the secretion of bile from the liver and gall bladder. Dandelion is a mild diuretic that flushes toxins from the liver, and it acts as a laxative too, so the entire digestive tract can work more efficiently. Along with dietary changes, these herbs can make a huge difference in the health and function of the liver and gall bladder. Hepatic herbs make good long-term tonics that can be enjoyed as cider vinegar salad dressing—just another name for medicine.

Extra-Strength Liver Cleanse

Yields 2 to 3 cups

2 tablespoons dried milk
  thistle seeds

¾ cup vodka

¼ cup water

2 tablespoons fresh
  burdock root, minced

2 tablespoons fresh yellow
  dock root, minced

2 tablespoons fresh
  dandelion root, minced

1 tablespoon dried nettle

1 teaspoon powdered
  turmeric

1½ cups apple cider
  vinegar, warmed

High in iron, this formula is a valuable tonic for liver tissue. Use freshly harvested and chopped roots whenever possible. Note: Do not take this formula if you are pregnant or nursing.

This is a two-part process. Place the milk thistle seeds in a 1-pint glass jar. Pour the vodka and water over them to ¼ inch of the rim; cap the jar and label it. Place the remaining herbs in a second 1-pint glass jar. Cover them with warm vinegar to the top of the jar; cap the jar and label it. (See chapter 4: Medicine-Making Methods for making a vinegar tincture) Allow both jars to steep for two weeks, preferably longer. Strain the liquids into one container and stir to combine. Take this preparation regularly, using the dosage guidelines on pages 287–90. Store the container with a plastic lid in a cool pantry or cabinet for up to two years.

Easy Salad Vinegar

Yields 3 cups

½ cup fresh burdock root,
  chopped

½ cup fresh yellow dock
  root, chopped

½ cup fresh dandelion
  root, chopped

¼ cup fresh parsley, chopped

3 cups apple cider vinegar

This tart and tasty vinegar can be used on fresh green salads, steamed broccoli, and sautéed turnip or collard greens—or however you like.

Follow the instructions in chapter 4: Medicine-Making Methods for making a vinegar tincture. Store the jar in the pantry for up to six months. When you're ready to make a salad dressing, add ⅓ cup vinegar to every ⅔ cup olive oil; season with salt, pepper, and fresh parsley to taste.

Directly connected to liver function is the urinary system. When healthy, the kidneys regularly pump urine out of the body and expel metabolic waste. When they are unhealthy, you feel a burning sensation or pain during urination, swelling, soreness, backache, headache, and often fever. If these symptoms persist, see a qualified health care practitioner. But at the first onset of symptoms, the following Urinary Tract Infection Tea can be what's needed to reverse the infection; calendula and yarrow kill bacteria, and dandelion "chauffeurs" them to the kidneys where they are needed. Marshmallow is a soothing demulcent, meaning it calms swelling and soothes inflamed tissues.

Urinary Tract Infection Tea

The urinary tract is a common location for infection, which can happen at any age. Babies and toddlers are prone to urinary tract infections (UTIs) simply because they put their hands in their mouths so frequently; teenagers, especially young women, can get this type of infection as a result of new hormone fluctuations. Adult women sometimes contract UTIs because of sexual activity, and menopausal women can get them from a decrease in progesterone and general vaginal dryness. This formula directs antibacterial herbs to the urinary tract where they can fight infection, soothe inflamed tissues, and heal.

Combine the herbs in a 1-quart glass jar. Pour enough boiling water over them to fill the jar. Steep for 5 to 8 minutes. The brew will be bitter and slightly thick; add honey to taste and drink 3 to 4 hot cups daily.

This bacteria-fighting tea can also be used effectively as a douche. Simply prepare it as a tea and follow the manufacturer's instructions for using douching equipment.

Yields 1 quart

2 tablespoons dried
  dandelion leaves
2 tablespoons dried
  calendula
2 tablespoons dried
  yarrow
1 tablespoon dried
  marshmallow
Honey

❧ Kidney Tonic Tea

Yields 1 quart

2 tablespoons dried
   dandelion leaves

1 tablespoon dried parsley

1 tablespoon dried plantain
   leaves

1 teaspoon dried red clover
   blossoms

1 teaspoon dried cleavers

1 teaspoon dried
   pipsissewa (optional)

Honey

If you are prone to kidney infections or are recovering from one, use this tea to nourish your urinary tract, keep the fluids flowing, and keep infection at bay. Visualize clean, clear tubing and free-flowing water. Note: Do not use this remedy if you are pregnant or breast-feeding.

Combine the herbs in a 1-quart glass jar. Pour enough boiling water over them to fill the jar. Steep for 5 to 8 minutes. The brew will be rather bitter; add honey to taste and drink 2 to 3 hot cups daily.

COLON

Ah, the digestive system! Nothing fascinated early herbalists and physicians as much as the digestive tract, with its yards of intestines, the colon, and the mysterious organs tucked safely in among them. And their ability to expel! Nineteenth-century physicians were well pleased when they could stimulate these and other organs to eliminate profusely: bowel movements were seen as a sure sign of recovery from illness and elimination of evil poisons, and the more explosive, the better.

Thankfully, we no longer seek to force this sort of evacuation, but we do value the digestive and elimination systems for removing what shouldn't stay in the body. There are many reasons the intestines and colon must work properly: metabolic waste removal is essential, or waste hormones and foodstuffs will be reabsorbed and recirculated, causing illness. Proper bowel movements remove hard, indigestible matter that would otherwise cause inflammation, pain, and swelling.

Some cultures, particularly the Native American nations, have routinely undergone cleanses to help their bodies maintain a steady ability to function. Sweat lodges (described in the next section) achieve similar physical results to those of the Danish and Swedish saunas, whereby the body is heated unnaturally high to produce a great deal of toxin-removing sweat, and plenty of fresh, clean water is taken in to replace it.

Attentive native nations were acutely aware of the many herbs available for causing the intestines and colon to cleanse themselves of matter. Today some clinicians offer colonics to remove waste matter from these organs, and others recommend home colonics as a safer and more comfortable process. But these procedures are invasive, costly, and certainly uncomfortable, regardless of whether you perform them in your own home or not. In my opinion, fresh herbs are superior, work quickly, naturally maintain the health of these hard-working organs, and pose fewer problems as long as they are used sparingly. *Note:* Do not use cleanses while you are pregnant or nursing.

Fiber Blend

Yields 2 cups

1 cup dried plantain seeds
1 cup whole flaxseeds
1 pinch powdered
cinnamon

For best results, the formulas in this section need to be taken with proper fiber so that when the bowels move, they have enough bulk to push waste products out. A deficiency in fiber will result in constipation—the bowels become stuck. Use this blend of herbs to maintain proper fiber if you're dieting or using one of the cleanses recommended here.

Harvest the plantain seeds from the wonderful weeds you've been selecting leaves from all summer—don't use store-bought psyllium. Store the herbs in the refrigerator until needed, and grind them together just before using. You may take 1 teaspoon in 1 cup of juice or water, but it's more enjoyable to sprinkle them on oatmeal, in breakfast cereal, and in smoothies. Or you can add a couple of teaspoons to muffins and breads.

Spring Cleansing Infusion

Yields 1 quart

2 parts fresh dandelion
  greens
2 parts fresh nettle leaves
1 part fresh, young, yellow
  dock root, cut into
  1-inch pieces
1 part fresh chicory greens
1 part fresh violet leaves
  and flowers
1 tablespoon dried licorice
  root, chopped
1 1-inch piece fresh ginger,
  chopped
1 quart boiling water
Honey

The herbs in this infusion are mildly laxative, nourishing, and bitter in order to stimulate digestive juices to flow and bowel movements to progress normally. Though infusions are usually made from dried herbs, these fresh, bright spring greens are too nourishing to be ignored after a cold, sluggish winter.

Clean and chop the fresh herbs and pack them tightly into a 1-pint glass jar. Add the yellow dock root, licorice root, and ginger and leave on top. Transfer the herbs from the jar to a deep soup pot, and pour the water over them. Cover the pot and steep for 15 to 20 minutes. The brew will be bitter; add honey to taste, and drink 3 to 5 hot cups daily for no more than 3 days.

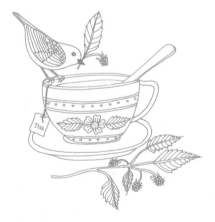

Summer Cleansing Infusion

The herbs used here are more readily available in summer after the early spring greens have disappeared. Motherwort and especially yarrow tend to be more warming bitters than the cool spring greens and help get the blood flowing. Calendula and yarrow are both antibacterial and support the overall cleansing effect of this formula.

Clean and chop all the herbs; pack them tightly into a 1-pint glass jar. Transfer them to a deep soup pot, and pour the water over them. Cover the pot and steep for 10 to 12 minutes. The brew will be bitter; add honey to taste, and drink 3 to 5 hot cups daily for no more than 3 days.

Yields 1 quart

2 parts fresh dandelion greens

2 parts fresh nettle greens

1 part fresh calendula flowers

1 part fresh red clover blossoms

½ part fresh motherwort leaves

½ part fresh yarrow leaves

1 quart boiling water

Honey

Fall and Winter Cleansing Decoction

In the fall, we tend to use the denser plant parts such as the roots, seeds, and berries. For this reason, this tea is really more of a decoction and requires a longer steeping time. Dandelion stays green well into the winter in most places, and it is just as valuable as it is in the spring for stimulating and supporting the liver.

Prepare this formula as a strong decoction (root brew), following the instructions in chapter 4: Medicine-Making Methods for making an herbal decoction. The brew will be bitter; add honey to taste, and drink 3 to 5 hot cups daily for no more than 3 days. You may also want to take the Fiber Blend described earlier during the same 3 days.

Yields 1 quart

1 cup fresh dandelion root, chopped

½ cup fresh yellow dock root, chopped

2 tablespoons dried elderberries

1 tablespoon dried licorice

1 1-inch piece fresh ginger, chopped

Honey

SWEATING

Our bodies sweat for many reasons: we're hot and the sweat beads on the skin and evaporates, which cools us off; we're nervous or scared, so our bodies produce adrenaline as part of the fight-or-flight response; we're overcoming a fever, and as it breaks, the body sweats (which cools us down and expels toxins). Along with many other reasons, the skin sweats because it is an organ of elimination, and many toxins and bacteria are removed through the pores.

A fever is the body's natural response to illness; though high fevers (above 100º F) should be addressed. Whether you are cleansing or trying to break a fever, the formulas in this section will encourage you to sweat. *Note:* Fevers above 103º F require immediate attention by a qualified health practitioner.

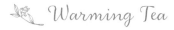 *Warming Tea*

Yields 1 quart

2 tablespoons dried ginger
  (not powder)
2 tablespoons dried licorice
2 tablespoons dried
  peppermint
1 teaspoon dried yarrow
Honey

Herbs that cause sweating are called diaphoretics, and in the right circumstances, they can be quite useful. Often employed for colds and flu to reduce fever, these herbs are also valuable during cleanses to stimulate blood flow to the periphery of the body and encourage sweating.

Prepare this formula as a decoction (root brew) by following the instructions in chapter 4: Medicine-Making Methods for making an herbal decoction. The brew will be bitter; add honey to taste, and drink it hot. Children should drink ½ cup every hour for a total of 1½ cups. To reduce fever or as a cleanse, adults should drink 1 cup every hour up to 3 cups per day.

Stimulating Massage Oil

Designed as an all-over body massage oil, this is equally as effective when rubbed on sore joints (see chapter 14: Aches and Pains), and it makes a wonderful gift. It brings blood flow to the surface of the skin and encourages the release of toxins through sweat. If you're using this during a cleanse, complete the massage by wrapping a hot towel around your body or applying a hot water bottle over a thin towel against the skin over the abdomen, lower back, or shoulders. After 30 minutes, rinse off in a cool shower. Note: Do not use this strong oil on young children.

Whisk all the ingredients together in a small jar or bowl. Use it as an all-over body rub, avoiding sensitive skin and the eyes.

Yields 1 cup

1 cup sweet almond, hemp, or jojoba oil

20 drops eucalyptus essential oil

20 drops Scotch pine essential oil

20 drops peppermint essential oil

10 drops clove essential oil

5 drops wintergreen or sweet birch essential oil

Deep-Cleansing Bath Salts

This is one of my favorite original formulas and has proven to be a wonderfully strong body-cleansing bath. The forest scent is invigorating, and the salts combine with the soothing glycerin to produce soft skin and relaxed muscles. Use solar-dried Dead Sea salts from a reputable source (see the Resources section at the end of this book for suppliers), and be sure to keep the salts and bathwater out of your eyes. Package the salts in a glass jar with a cork.

Follow the instructions in chapter 4: Medicine-Making Methods for making bath salts. When drawing your bath, sprinkle 3 to 5 tablespoons of the salt mixture under hot running water and allow it to dissolve. Get a thermos of cool water and have it tubside; be sure to drink at least a quart of water during the bath. For maximum benefit, massage your body while in the bath to invigorate the muscles and encourage blood flow while the body is hot. This type of bath is not recommended for children under twelve.

Yields approximately 4 cups

1 cup Dead Sea salts

2 cups Epsom salts

½ cup baking soda (sodium bicarbonate)

2 tablespoons vegetable glycerin

40 drops basil essential oil

40 drops balsam fir essential oil

BLOOD "CLEANSER"

Springtime is a wonderful season for cleansing the body. Of course, we're not dirty, but after a long cold winter, our internal systems may be a bit sluggish and in need of freedom from all those thick casseroles and hearty meat dishes. Even Mother Nature accommodates us: the new green leaves sprouting forth at this time are bitter and sometimes tangy, perfect for stimulating the liver and the production of bile from the gall bladder. Bitters have long been a traditional remedy in the spring, especially in the southern Appalachian mountains where I grew up. It was common to see people out in their fields before the first plow, harvesting fresh new mustard greens (called "creasies") and dandelion greens.

Use the Delicious Spring Salad and the Spring Bitters Tincture on a daily basis for two to four weeks during the spring; also, simplify your meals and begin to wean your body from heavier winter foods. Increase exercise levels, walk more, wake earlier, and feel your body growing stronger and livelier.

Delicious Spring Salad

Harvest the wild weeds while the leaves are shorter than 3 to 4 inches.

Yields 2 to 4 servings

For the Salad
A combination of any of the following to equal 2 to 4 large handfuls:
Purslane (*portulaca*)
Dandelion leaves

Mint leaves
Poke leaf
Plantain leaves
Yellow dock leaves
Chicory leaves
Wood sorrel
Early thyme
Oregano

Wild lettuce
Sweet Cicely
Watercress

For the Dressing
½ cup extra virgin olive oil
3 tablespoons to ¼ cup apple cider, red or white wine, balsamic vinegar, or freshly squeezed lemon juice
Salt and pepper to taste

Toss the greens into a large bowl. Combine all of the ingredients for the dressing in a jar. Drizzle the dressing over the greens and eat as a salad, or pack into a whole-grain sandwich with chopped dried tomatoes. Store the dressing in a glass jar in the refrigerator for up to 8 months.

Spring Asparagus Meal

Harvest any of these shoots judiciously and follow the traditional herbalist's gathering mantra: Take only one plant for every ten you see.

Clean the shoots, then chop them coarsely into 1-inch lengths. Place them in a steamer. Steam lightly for 5 to 10 minutes, or until the shoots are tender but still retain their bright green color. Sprinkle them with lemon juice or vinegar and salt to taste, and serve them as a side vegetable.

Yields 2 to 4 servings

A combination of any
    of the following to
    make up 2 to 4 large
    handfuls:
Solomon's seal shoots
Cattail shoots
Wild asparagus shoots
Japanese knotweed shoots

Spring Bitters Tincture

Bitters are traditionally used to stimulate the digestive juices and are a favorite springtime indulgence. It's important to taste the bitter flavor of this tincture, so allow it to sit on your tongue for a few moments—after all, proper digestion begins in the mouth.

Combine the herbs in a 1-pint glass jar, and follow the instructions in chapter 4: Medicine-Making Methods for making a vinegar tincture. Sprinkle the liquid on salads, or take it medicinally—5 to 15 drops 3 times daily, preferably before meals.

Yields 2 cups

¼ cup fresh dandelion
    leaves and root, minced
¼ cup fresh yellow dock
    leaves and root, minced
¼ cup fresh watercress
    or other early mustard
    greens, minced
1 tablespoon fresh, young
    yarrow leaves, minced
1½ cups apple cider vinegar

ECZEMA AND PSORIASIS

Though many people regard eczema and psoriasis strictly as annoying skin conditions, herbal heritage teaches that they are actually the result of an inner imbalance, usually in the liver. For this reason, remedies for eczema and psoriasis are placed in this chapter on cleansing and detox. The skin eruptions (inflammation, rashes, and itching) are merely symptoms of a much deeper imbalance that needs to be addressed with herbs that detoxify the overloaded gastrointestinal, hepatic, nervous, and sometimes reproductive systems. The true cause of eczema often lies in the digestive tract; you will need to examine liver health and explore food allergies. For remedies addressing other skin wounds or complaints, see chapter 11: Healing Wounds or chapter 17: Beauty, Skin, and Body Care.

As an herbalist, I frequently receive questions about and requests for eczema remedies. I've seen many ugly rashes: eczema, psoriasis, yeast infections, burns, allergic reactions, poison ivy, or any other manner of skin reactions. I recognize the fear and concern of those dealing with these bizarre and abnormal irritations, especially when the eruptions occur frequently and "for no apparent reason." Some are severe and can appear in alarming places, such as the eyelids. I always recommend a visit to a trusted health care practitioner, but I also say that people have traditionally and successfully used herbs to address and relieve these problems.

Eczema and psoriasis begin inside the body but express themselves through the skin (and other organs). Eczema is characterized by oozing, red, blisterlike pustules that itch and often crust over. They are usually found in the warm, moist areas of the body: in the creases of the elbows and knees, the folds of the neck, or the navel. The hands will often display the typical eczema rash. Eczema is thought to have two causes: the most common is an allergy to an external irritant such as industrial solvents, dyes, soaps and shampoos, or heat; the second is diet. Many people clear up eczema by removing dairy, wheat, or sugar from their diet.

Psoriasis, on the other hand, is characterized by gray, dry, nonitchy scales usually found on the dry, bony parts of the body—elbows, kneecaps, or ribs. Something triggers the skin cells to proliferate more quickly than they can be shed. Most remedies, therefore, involve changing diet, moisturizing the area, and gently scrubbing to remove the scales.

If you or a loved one has been diagnosed with eczema, psoriasis, or a yeast infection, or if you believe a rash may be an allergic reaction to environmental pollutants or a particular food, follow these guidelines.

- Relax. Many people experience rashes as a reaction to stress, which can trigger hormone production and responses from the pituitary and adrenal glands. These responses are the body's protection from perceived attack and are meant to keep us safe, but they often go ignored and lead to chronic stress and the expression of toxins through the skin. Try taking a salt bath (see the recipe for Deep-Cleansing Bath Salts earlier in this chapter) or use the Lavender Massage Oil recipe in chapter 14: Aches and Pains.
- Adjust your diet. Many rashes are the body's reaction to eating foreign or uncooperative foods, and dairy is a prime culprit. Yeast (a common fungus, *Candida albicans*) thrives on dairy, sugars, and refined grains such as wheat. Many rashes clear up quickly once these foods are removed from the diet.
- Take acidophilus, especially *Lactobacillus acidophilus*. These probiotics protect the gastrointestinal tract by providing living organisms that normally inhabit the body, and they improve digestion and liver function.
- Care for your liver. As a detoxifying organ (along with the skin, kidneys, lungs, colon, and lymph system), the liver is tasked with removing harmful substances from the body. For this reason, hepatic (liver-healing) herbs such as those in the following recipes are useful.

Alterative Internal Tincture for Eczema

Yields 2 to 3 cups

¼ cup fresh burdock root, chopped

¼ cup fresh yellow dock root, chopped

¼ cup fresh dandelion root, chopped

¼ cup fresh dandelion leaves, chopped

¼ cup fresh red clover blossoms, chopped

¼ cup fresh calendula, chopped

3 to 4 tablespoons fresh mint, minced

2 cups apple cider vinegar

½ cup water

¼ cup grain alcohol such as vodka or brandy

I've seen wonderful results with this and the alterative lotion that follows. This formula is for internal use, and the lotion is for external; used in tandem, they combine antifungal, antibacterial, alterative, and soothing herbs to alleviate itching, speed the healing of skin tissues, alter the body's responses to allergens, and fight fungal and bacterial infections. Along with dietary adjustments to remove allergens (especially dairy and wheat), these formulas create a strong foundation for eradicating eczema and psoriasis.

Follow the instructions in chapter 4: Medicine-Making Methods for making a vinegar tincture, adding the grain alcohol after the vinegar has cooled. Follow the dosage guidelines on page 288 for adult chronic conditions. Use the tincture for three weeks on, then one week off. Repeat the cycle as needed.

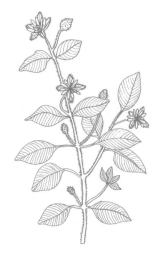

Alterative Lotion for Eczema and Psoriasis

This is the external lotion counterpart to the preceding tincture. Both calendula and pau d'arco are traditional remedies to address yeast infections, and black cumin seed, red raspberry, and kukui nut oil (Aleurites moluccana) are traditionally used to relieve eczema and skin rashes. This antifungal recipe is moisturizing and works quickly to lift psoriasis scales and clear the skin of eczema and yeast infections. Be sure to follow a diet free of sugars, coffee, and yeasty breads for best effect. This is a liquidy lotion, and it will not get thick like a hand lotion. Thin and pleasant, it soaks into the skin easily. Shake well before using, apply it with a cotton ball, and avoid the eyes.

Soak the pau d'arco and calendula in the witch hazel in a glass quart jar as if making a tincture. If you are using dried herbs, use a ratio of one part herb to four parts witch hazel. Let this steep in a cool, dark closet for two weeks, shaking occasionally. Strain the liquid and add the oils and aloe vera juice. Whisk until the lotion reaches the desired consistency; add the sweet orange extract one drop at a time for scent. Pour it into a clean bottle, and label it "for external use only." Stored in the pantry, this lotion will keep up to three years. Shake well before using.

Yields approximately 2 cups

½ cup dried or fresh calendula flowers

½ cup dried pau d'arco herb

1 cup distilled witch hazel

2 tablespoons black cumin seed oil (*Nigella sativa*)

2 tablespoons red raspberry or kukui nut oil

2 tablespoons aloe vera juice

Few drops sweet orange extract

Eczema Itch Relief

Chickweed is a sweet, trailing little herb that grows in cold, clear creeks and rich woodlands. It is easy to harvest, is a traditional "specific" for soothing itchy skin, and can be used safely at any age—even with infants. If you can't find fresh chickweed, substitute dried calendula flowers.

Place the herbs in a 1-pint glass jar and pour the liquid over them. Steep in a dark cabinet for two weeks, shaking occasionally. Strain the liquid, pour it into a clean bottle, and label it "for external use only." Apply it with a cotton ball as needed, keeping away from the eyes.

Yields 2 cups

1 packed cup fresh chickweed herb, minced

1 packed cup fresh dandelion leaves, minced

2 cups witch hazel or apple cider vinegar

Easy Calendula-Beeswax Salve

Yields 1 cup

1 cup packed fresh
   calendula flowers (or ¼
   cup dried)

1 cup olive or canola oil

¼ cup beeswax

Used internally, calendula acts as a strong antifungal; used externally in this antifungal salve, it is also extremely moisturizing. Many people report great relief when soothing their itchy skin with this rich, honey-scented beeswax salve.

In a sauce pot, heat the flowers and oil together on very low heat for 20 minutes, stirring frequently. Strain the liquid and return the oil to the pot. Melt the beeswax into the oil; when it is thoroughly mixed and pour the salve into a glass jar. Apply this salve to the skin frequently.

Chapter Sixteen

—◦◦◦—

MIND AND SPIRIT

One of the reasons so many of us love herbs is because they are functional and have medicinal effects on the body. They heal our wounds and repair tissues. But they do much more than that: green plants gift us with something almost imperceptible, something more spiritual than physical.

We don't need a scientist telling us about positive ions to know that a walk through a rich forest is a healing experience. Ions or not, the trees are therapists in their own right, as are the herbs underfoot and the amazing connecting fungi that hold the forest together. This is why we desire to be in nature when we're sad or upset; we burst from our homes and escape to the woods, the meadows, the lake, the ocean, the sanctuaries that are a blessing to us and are ready when we need them. The plants that grow in these sanctuaries (and the weeds that grow by our own backdoors) harbor chemicals that affect the nervous system, but even more than that, they harbor a universal spirit every bit as wonderful as any we can imagine. There is a magnificent wisdom inherent in nature, the planet's expression of beauty; as Ralph Waldo Emerson said, "Earth laughs in flowers." Laughter is a harbor, a place of refuge and protection when our spirits are confused or threatened.

British herbalist Anne McIntyre told me it doesn't matter how you use a plant as long as you connect with it. We can pursue our understanding of phytochemicals until the cows come home, but we may never truly learn how plants such as lemon balm, roses, and ashwaghanda (*Withania somnifera*) perform their magic on the nervous system and brain tissues. But they do. They have for millennia and have been revered as tonic herbs, sustaining herbs, life-enhancing herbs, and even heal-all remedies. Plants, simply by *being*, deserve our respect and appreciation. They simply are. And they are beautiful.

Over millennia, people have realized that herbs, among many other green friends, heal the spirit as well as the body, and we treasure them in our pursuit of longevity, understanding, and wisdom.

ANXIETY

Whether you're a nervous Nellie or are going through a trying time in your life that brings on anxiety, tremors, difficulty sleeping, shortness of breath, or difficulty concentrating, you can call on herbs to help you find your balance. The herbs in this section have been used with success for many years to center thoughts and reduce the body's reaction to stress. Herbalists affectionately call them "adaptogens," as they help us adapt. They can't take away the stressful situation, but they can help your central nervous system react in a healthy way, allowing you to process information accurately and communicate with others with confidence and strength.

Ancient Flower Healer Tea

Yields 1 quart

2 tablespoons dried gotu kola leaves

2 tablespoons dried lemon balm

1 tablespoon dried red clover blossoms

1 tablespoon dried rose petals

These herbs tend to bring blood flow to the brain and are frequently used to improve concentration and memory. They are also nourishing to the central nervous system and make a delightfully delicious tea.

Combine the herbs in a 1-quart glass jar, and cover them with enough boiling water to fill the jar. Steep for 10 to 12 minutes, tightly covered; if you want a very strong brew, steep for an hour. Strain the tea and drink it freely. Generally, this formula should be taken consistently 2 to 3 times daily for two to three weeks or longer. Be sure to take advantage of your other healing sources: friends, exercise, yoga, good foods, meditation, and adequate sleep.

MILD DEPRESSION

Certain herbs have been clinically proven to address mild depression; sales of Saint-John's-wort have surpassed sales of Prozac in Germany. As a flower and therefore a completely natural remedy, Saint-John's-wort offers great benefits with fewer side effects, though some people experience photosensitivity while taking this herb. Of course, take any form of severe depression very seriously and consult a qualified health care practitioner.

In addition to the following formulas, pay special attention to your liver if you are depressed and even consider doing a toxin cleanse, since a healthy liver benefits all the body's systems. You may also want to monitor hormonal changes, as some depression can be linked to cyclical hormonal activity that can be addressed with diet and/or herbal remedies (see the Wild Yam PMS Jam formula in chapter 7: Especially for Women).

Mood Mend Tincture

I developed this formula using the "gladdening herbs," as they are affectionately called. Beneficial for children, teens, and adults alike, these anxiety-relieving herbs are renowned for lifting the spirits and improving outlook on life.

Combine the herbs in a 1-quart glass jar and cover them with the alcohol, glycerin, and water. Follow the instructions in chapter 4: Medicine-Making Methods for making an alcohol tincture. Use this tincture consistently 2 to 3 times daily for two to three months for best results.

Yields 2 cups

1 cup packed fresh lemon balm, chopped
1 cup packed fresh Saint-John's-wort flowers and leaves, chopped
½ cup fresh borage flowers
½ cup fresh rose petals
Equal parts grain alcohol, vegetable glycerin, and distilled water

Children's Little Lift Tea

Yields 1 quart

2 tablespoons dried lemon
balm

1 tablespoon dried lemon
verbena

1 tablespoon dried rose
petals

1 tablespoon dried borage
flowers and/or leaves

This is a delicious lemony tea to lift the spirits and ease stress, confusion, and scattered thoughts.

Combine the herbs in a 1-quart glass jar, and pour enough boiling water over them to fill the jar. Steep for 8 to 10 minutes, strain the liquid, and sweeten with honey if desired. Let the child drink the tea warm or cold. This infusion makes a wonderfully soothing drink at the end of a hot summer day. It also makes a delicious hot beverage as an off-to-school mind opener in the morning.

GRIEF AND LOSS

Sadness and grief can actually bring on illness. The loss of a beloved friend, relative, or pet; the loss of a job, home, or endeavor; or even the empathy surrounding the sadness experienced by someone else are enough to cause nausea, headaches, and lethargy. Grief is a profound response that most people associate with the heart, though its causes are often spiritual or formed somewhere in the brain. Flowers and herbs create a wonderful support system during these trying times. In addition to the herbal remedies in this section, flower essences for grief and sadness include sugar maple, hawthorn, and purple clematis. Flower essences are energetic, meaning they work via spiritual channels little understood by modern science. Since they contain no plant chemicals (as herbal concentrates do), flower essences gently nourish and strengthen our emotions, as if the plant itself is acting as our personal guidance counselor. (Many flower essences can be found at your local health food store; see also the Resources section at the end of this book for recommended producers.)

FLOWER ESSENCES

Because of their beauty, color, and fragrance, flowers have been humanity's choice comfort medicine for millennia. Their commercial popularity is credited to Dr. Edward Bach (1886–1936), an English surgeon and immunologist who abandoned conventional medicine to pursue natural and noninvasive therapies. He taught us how to capture the allure of flowers in liquid form and how to use it for emotional therapy. Today, healing arts practitioners love flower essences for their ability to gently center the consciousness and clear emotions.

Flower essences differ from the tinctures described in this book in many ways. First, while tinctures are concentrated extracts of plants—high in phytochemicals such as essential oils, acids, alcohols, and glycosides—a flower essence captures the "vibrational essence" or energy of the plant, delivering its medicine spiritually or energetically rather than physically. Second, though tinctures and flower essences are generally preserved with alcohol (flower essences almost always with brandy), their methods of preparation differ. Herbs for a tincture are steeped in alcohol and water for a length of time, but flowers need not touch the liquid in which their essence is captured. Some herbalists may dip the flower into the liquid to make its essence, while others simply place the bowl of liquid nearby. Third, while tinctures are often "put up" by the moon, using lunar gravitational influence to enhance the strength of the tincture, flower essences are considered to actually contain lunar energy.

Falling somewhere between homeopathic remedies and concentrated herbal tinctures, flower essences affect our emotions, which can best be demonstrated, in my opinion, in animals. While the human mind may balk at the value of flower essences and thereby cause the treatment to fail, animals have no such qualms. The plant world has many mysteries we have yet to uncover, and working with flowers on an energetic level to treat our emotions is at once charming and effective.

Rose-Hawthorn Formula

Hawthorn is a long-trusted heart herb often used for cardiac support and to reduce high blood pressure, but many people turn to it during times of stress, sadness, and even depression. Roses are considered the flower of rebirth, healing, love, and beauty, and simply being near them and inhaling their miraculous scent can improve your spirits.

Yields 2 cups

1 cup fresh hawthorn
    flowers and leaves (or ¼
    cup dried)
1 cup fresh rose petals (or
    ¼ cup dried)
1 cup grain alcohol such as
    vodka or brandy
½ cup vegetable glycerin
½ cup water

As a Tincture

Combine the herbs in a 1-quart glass jar, and follow the instructions in chapter 4: Medicine-Making Methods for making an alcohol tincture. Take 5 to 20 drops 3 times daily.

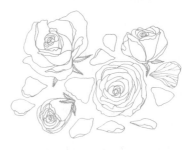

Yields 1 quart

3 tablespoons dried
    hawthorn flowers and
    leaves
2 tablespoons dried rose
    petals
Honey

As a Tea

Combine the herbs in a 1-quart glass jar, and cover them with enough boiling water to fill the jar. Follow the instructions in chapter 4: Medicine-Making Methods for making an herbal infusion. Sweeten with honey to taste and drink 3 to 4 warm cups daily.

As an Oil

Follow the instructions in chapter 4: Medicine-Making Methods for making an herbal oil. Apply the oil to your temples, wrists, neck, and over your heart as desired.

Yields 2 cups

1 cup fresh hawthorn
flowers and leaves (or ¼
cup dried)
1 cup fresh rose petals (or
¼ cup dried)
2 cups sweet almond oil

As a Salve

Using the 2 cups oil from the preceding instructions, follow the instructions in chapter 4: Medicine-Making Methods for making an herbal salve, using ½ cup chopped beeswax. Apply the creamy salve to your temples, wrists, neck, and over your heart as desired.

Yields 2 cups

Vineyard Summer Lemon Tea

Bright, citrusy, lemony flavors wake up the spirit and open your eyes. These herbs all release their fresh citrus scents when made into a fragrant infusion: drink it hot for a soothing, warming feeling in the heart, or drink it cold on hot days to revive the spirit and boost your energy.

Follow the instructions in chapter 4: Medicine-Making Methods for making an herbal infusion. Drink this tea freely, hot or iced.

Yields 1 quart

2 tablespoons dried lemon
balm
2 tablespoons dried
lemongrass
2 tablespoons dried lemon
verbena
1 teaspoon dried alfalfa
1 teaspoon fresh lemon
peel (or ¼ teaspoon
dried)

INSOMNIA

Being unable to sleep is devastating to the psyche, which feels unable to control the body and at a loss for how to proceed with something that should be happening. This invites frustration and, of course, prolongs the inability to sleep.

Thankfully, we are blessed with many sedative herbs—plants that make us sleepy. Often these herbs depress the central nervous system, allowing the body to shut down for the night; sometimes they simply help the nervous system deal with stress and anxiety and process these emotions in a healthy way.

There are several tricks to helping your body relax:

- Meditate. Envision your body relaxing from your head down your neck and spine, and finally through your hips, legs, and feet. Let each part of your body sink into the mattress, and take your time with this meditation. Envision yourself at a lulling spot—on a raft on a lake, on the deck of a meandering ship, on a bed of moss in the cool of the woods.
- Thank the universe for everything. This will often bring you to a stumbling block: you'll be thankful for everything until you get to something that bothers you. Likely, the thought of this thing or person is what's keeping you awake. Be thankful anyway. Let it go.
- Indulge in a hot bath before bed. This is especially useful for children who may be worried about something the next day.

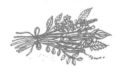

Children's Sleepytime Tonic

For children who can't sleep, try the preceding methods along with this tincture and a cup of Hot Chamomile-Rose Tea (the recipe follows). With the combination of a warm bath, hot tea, lulling fragrances, and soothing herbs, a tiny dose of this tincture is generally sufficient to help your child relax and sleep through the night.

Follow the instructions in chapter 4: Medicine-Making Methods for making an alcohol tincture, using a 1-pint glass jar in place of the 1-quart jar. Give your child ½ teaspoon an hour before bed and another ½ teaspoon at bedtime, preferably in a cup of Hot Chamomile-Rose Tea.

Yields 2 cups

½ cup fresh chamomile
½ cup fresh rose petals
½ cup fresh wild lettuce
1 cup grain alcohol such as
    vodka or brandy
¾ cup water
¼ cup vegetable glycerin

Hot Chamomile-Rose Tea

Chamomile is world-renowned as a soporific herb, and it is usually enjoyed at bedtime. As a mild bitter, it enhances proper digestion, soothes the stomach, calms the nerves, and acts as a rather powerful sedative. Combined with roses, which soothe the central nervous system and ease heartache (literally and figuratively), chamomile is a wonderful remedy for insomnia.

Combine the herbs in a 1-quart glass jar, and cover them with enough boiling water to fill the jar. Steep for 5 to 8 minutes and strain. Drink this lovely tea unsweetened and hot before bedtime, taking slow sips and thinking restful thoughts.

Yields 1 quart

3 tablespoons dried
    chamomile flowers
1 tablespoon dried rose
    petals

Sleep Ease Tincture for Adults

Yields 2 cups

¼ cup dried hops

¼ cup dried chamomile

¼ cup dried passionflower

1 cup grain alcohol (such as
vodka, brandy, rum, or
port wine)

1 cup water

Hops *refers to the fruit of* Humulus lupulus, *a climbing vine. The dangling, flowerlike fruits produce a yellow, dusty resin that stains hands yellow. Hops combines well with other sedative herbs, such as chamomile and passionflower, to create an effective remedy for insomnia.*

Follow the instructions in chapter 4: Medicine-Making Methods for making an alcohol tincture, using a 1-pint glass jar instead of the 1-quart jar. Take ½ teaspoon an hour before bedtime and another ½ teaspoon at bedtime, preferably in Hot Chamomile-Rose Tea (described previously). Keep the tincture on your bedside table and take another ½ teaspoonful if you wake during the night; getting up can wake you even more.

Rest Well Tea

Yields 1 quart

2 tablespoons dried
chamomile flowers

2 tablespoons dried
passionflowers

1 tablespoon dried Saint-
John's-wort herb

1 teaspoon dried rose
petals

This is a lovely tea that acts as a sedative without leaving you feeling drugged or knocked out. It's a satisfying bedtime brew, delightful for children and adults alike. Saint-John's-wort is high in tryptophan, which can increase serotonin levels in the brain, improving neurotransmitter function that can help relieve insomnia.

Combine the herbs in a 1-quart glass jar. Pour enough boiling water over them to fill the jar. Brew according to the instructions in chapter 4: Medicine-Making Methods for making an herbal tea. Drink 1 cup an hour before bedtime and another cup at bedtime.

ATTENTION DEFICIT/HYPERACTIVITY DISORDER, LACK OF FOCUS, AND HYPERACTIVITY

Not all brains work alike. Some are quiet and studious; others are loud and full of movement. They may all be bright, loving, creative, and curious, but their method of taking external signals and converting them to something useful may be quite different. Children with loud brains that encourage quickly moving bodies often struggle in America's public school system, where they are taught to be quiet, still, and "absorbent." Children diagnosed with attention deficit disorder (ADD) or attention-deficit/hyperactivity disorder (ADHD)—or simply labeled hyperactive, inattentive, or spirited—often tap their pencils, their feet, and their hands; make "bop" sounds with their lips; get up and down frequently; and have trouble being still and silent. In both teachers and children, frustration levels can run high.

Parent advocates have useful dietary and herbal protocols at their disposal. Small changes can lead to a satisfying and fulfilling life (and school experience) for children and their families:

- Remove foods high in salicylates from your child's diet. Normally salicylates provide pain relief and are used in herbal analgesic formulas, but they pose a problem for certain children. Salicylate-containing foods include caffeinated beverages, honey, yeast (breads), and most fruit juices. Even peppermint flavoring and nuts can have a high salicylate content, which can interfere with the brain's ability to self-regulate in individuals with ADD/ADHD.
- Don't allow your child to eat foods containing monosodium glutamate (MSG) or artificially flavored or artificially colored foods.
- Encourage your child to eat cabbage, slaw, sauerkraut, celery, chives, peas and legumes, fresh sprouts, potatoes, and garlic.

The Clarity Fountain

The herbs in this formula have been used for centuries to help the brain and body cope with excessive input, mild depression, and a barrage of external stimuli. Lemon balm (Melissa officinalis) has long been hailed as an aid for those suffering from inattention and lack of focus. According to internationally renowned herbalist and medical doctor Tieraona Low Dog, lemon balm affects the limbic-hippocampal area of the brain and can "filter out" external stimuli so the brain can concentrate. Ginkgo stimulates blood flow to the brain, and Saint-John's-wort eases anxiety. Use this formula for children, teens, and adults who suffer from ADHD.

Yields 2 cups

¾ cup fresh lemon balm

¾ cup fresh Saint-John's-wort

¼ cup dried ginkgo

1 cup brandy

1 cup water

As a Tincture

Follow the instructions in chapter 4: Medicine-Making Methods for making an alcohol tincture. For children who are old enough, administering the dose alone can improve confidence and create a feeling of satisfaction and control. Take 30 to 40 drops 2 to 3 times daily in water or tea.

Yields 1 quart

2 tablespoons dried lemon balm

2 tablespoons dried Saint-John's-wort

1 tablespoon dried ginkgo

As a Tea

Combine the herbs in a 1-quart glass jar. Pour enough boiling water over them to fill the jar. Steep for 5 to 8 minutes. Strain the liquid and keep it in a thermos for cold weather, or ice it during hot weather (it tastes delicious both ways). Let your child drink it freely—at least 2 to 3 cups daily.

MEMORY PROBLEMS

Certain herbs stimulate blood flow to the brain. Ginkgo is renowned for this and has become a favorite herb of seniors, although anyone can use it. Lemon balm, because of its ability to aid mental clarity and focus, is often used in memory formulas. Gotu kola is a lovely herb with an affinity for the mind and can be eaten as a salad herb or used in formulas. Other helpful herbs include damiana, rosemary, hawthorn berry, motherwort, borage and bugleweed, many of which are also used in cardiac tonics (see chapter 12: Happy Heart).

Memory Boost Tincture

Use this formula during test week (the week prior and the week of), during exams, when training for a new job, during menopause, or any other time your brain feels scattered or you wish to improve your memory. Also try fun mind games and brain teasers that strengthen your thought processes and "grease" the mental machinery.

Follow the instructions in chapter 4: Medicine-Making Methods for making an alcohol tincture, using a 1-pint glass jar instead of the 1-quart jar. Bottle, label, and store in the pantry. Use the dosage guidelines on pages 287–90.

Yields 2 cups

¼ cup dried ginkgo

2 tablespoons fresh lemon balm

2 tablespoons fresh gotu kola (or 1 tablespoon dried)

1 tablespoon dried damiana

1 cup brandy

1 cup water

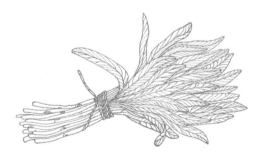

One of my favorite ways to use plants is in ceremony. We all participate in ceremonies and ritual traditions: blowing out candles at a birthday party, brewing a morning cup of coffee, bringing our child's teacher a holiday gift. When my family moved into our house, my friend Mary came over with a bowl, a lighter, and a bundle of dried sage to clear the energies and bless the new house. It made a world of difference.

Plants engage in our lives in myriad ways. Our custom of sending flowers to funerals recognizes on a deep level the special emotional connection we share with flowers. We have them at weddings, not simply because they are beautiful, but also because they represent beauty and love and permanence. We build our homes with wood, not only because wood is a superb building material, but because it connects us with the power and long-standing patience of trees.

Include plants in your meditations and prayers. Get to know them. Many herbalists, such as Eliot Cowan, call this "plant spirit medicine" and encourage the connection with plants on a spiritual level to speed healing. I couldn't agree more, and I believe your own intuitive connections will show you how to use plants, which parts, and for what (emotional as well as physical) purposes.

For example, over the course of a meditative year, I hiked many trails across the Ridge Mountains of North Carolina and connected with a number of plants not generally considered medicinal. But I discovered remedies that operate on an energetic level, such as creeping phlox (instructive for creating your future and manifesting life changes); hemlock (for reducing feelings of aloneness and separation); white oak (for relieving stress), and trillium (for promoting unity and completion).

Intuition is a powerful tool available to anyone willing to listen to his or her inner voice with patience and trust. Harnessing this inner wisdom can bring fulfillment, wellness, and peace.

TRANSITION AND CHANGES

Transitions are a part of life; birth marks the beginning of what will be a life of transition and changes. The challenge is to embrace each of them with grace and humor so that we may grow a little each time. Ancient men and women looked to Hecate, goddess of the crossroads, to guide them through both positive and negative changes, including marriages, deaths, pilgrimages, children leaving home, war, lost love, and even the natural process of aging. To them, Hecate represented the strength to let go of the past and embrace the future, to allow nature to shed old skin to reveal new skin beneath the surface. Pivotal crossroads allow us the frightening freedom to choose our future direction; sometimes we wish someone else would do it for us. The courage to make these decisions marks the growth of wisdom and the ability to self-direct. This is what life is about.

Crossroads Tea

This tea is a ceremonial recognition of changes and crossroads. It is deeply grounding and centering. Brew it with love and strength in your heart, and share a cup with a loved one.

Place the ginger in a pan with the water. Bring to a simmer and heat for 5 to 8 minutes. Add the violet flowers, stir, and remove from the heat. Cover tightly and steep 5 to 8 minutes. Strain the tea and sweeten as desired.

Yields 1 quart

2 tablespoons dried ginger, chopped

1 quart water

2 tablespoons dried violet flowers

✤ Hecate's Heart

Yields 2 cups

½ cup fresh mugwort
   leaves
½ cup fresh packed chicory
   flowers
½ cup fresh hawthorn
   leaves, flowers, or
   berries
2 to 3 drops Eastern
   hemlock flower essence
   (optional)
1 cup brandy or port wine
1 cup water

This is a tincture for those times when a little extra emotional strength is needed.

Follow the instructions in chapter 4: Medicine-Making Methods for making an alcohol tincture, adding the flower essence as you bottle the strained tincture. Take 3 to 5 drops on the tongue or in tea, as needed every hour throughout the day.

✤ Sanctuary Balm

Yields approximately ½ cup

1 tablespoon dried angelica
   root
4 tablespoons coconut oil
   or cocoa butter
Rose essential oil
Flower essences (such as
   lavender, scarlet basil,
   sunflower, ironweed,
   rose, or red clover)

This creamy ointment is a ceremonial balm for special occasions. Scent it with whatever flower essences you desire.

Without heating, use a spoon to blend the angelica root into the oil or butter, mashing until all the roots are covered. Let the mixture sit one whole moon cycle (full to full is best).

In a small saucepan, melt the oil over gentle heat until the roots can be strained out. Strain and return the oil or butter to the pan. Add the essential oil and flower essences, and quickly pour it into the container of your choice—something lovely like a ceramic bowl with a cork lid or a glass container with a glass lid. Rub the balm gently into your temples and wrists or over your heart.

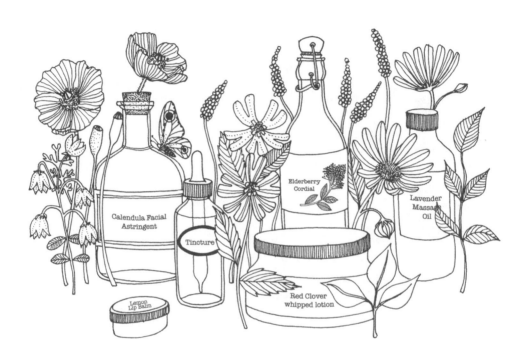

Calendula Facial
Astringent

Tincture

Lemon
Lip Balm

Elderberry
Cordial

Red Clover
whipped lotion

Lavender
Massage
Oil

Part Five

RECIPES FOR
HERBAL DELIGHTS

In my house, we may not have anything to eat, but we have flowers.

—Doña Enriqueta Contreras

Chapter Seventeen

SKIN AND BODY CARE

We know that what's on the inside is what counts, but beauty on the outside is also important. It's what signals that we are fulfilled, joyful, and happy with life. Glowing skin is not the result of cosmetics (though the toners and moisturizers in this chapter can help rejuvenate tired skin), but it is the culmination of a life well lived, a spirit well fed.

As the skin is our largest organ (and an organ of elimination, at that), it needs constant care and nurturing for its continued health. Your skin says a lot about you (as does the health of your hair): Is it tired, dry, and papery? Greasy, sallow, and pitted? These conditions indicate an imbalance in your body that can be addressed by any of the remedies outlined in the previous chapters. These conditions (and usually the imbalances that cause them) are reversible and can always be resolved using natural methods that heighten your energy and nourish your life.

The skin, hair, and body treatments that follow can be enjoyed by most teens, men, and women (though specific body care formulas for men and women are found in chapter 7: Especially for Women and chapter 8: Especially for Men). Let the making of these remedies be fun activities that you do frequently, as these products tend to have short shelf lives. Use them often and enjoy your radiant (and healthy) skin and hair.

ACNE

Acne is partly a skin condition but mostly the result of a hormonal condition. Both teens and adults experience it when undergoing hormonal changes. The pituitary gland is a complex organ that can be balanced using herbs such as chaste tree berry and red clover, but there are also surface remedies that can address skin problems on the spot. The remedies that follow include both external and internal options.

Cooling Acne Wash

Yields 1 cup

½ cup fresh burdock root, chopped

½ cup fresh calendula petals

¼ cup fresh lavender flowers

1 cup witch hazel

1 tablespoon apple cider vinegar

This wash is refreshing and great for hot, inflamed, blistering acne.

Place all the plant material in a 1-pint glass jar, and cover it with witch hazel and vinegar. Cap the jar, label it, and let it steep in a dark cabinet overnight or up to two weeks. Strain the liquid well through cheesecloth, and pour it into a clean bottle. Use a cotton ball to apply it to acne, pimples, rashes, and blisters. Refrigerate it for a cooling effect.

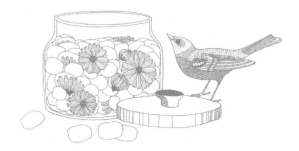

Mullein Acne Soother

This is a soothing astringent for broken, weepy acne and for skin that has become rough or pitted. Use this compress for acute flare-ups or each evening for stubborn, chronic conditions until the skin clears.

Follow the instructions in chapter 4: Medicine-Making Methods for making a compress. Be sure to strain the mullein through several layers of cheesecloth to remove tiny hairs.

This soothing compress is best applied while you are reclining and relaxing. Allow the first cloth to remain on your face as long as it feels comfortable and is warm, 7 to 8 minutes. Remove it and replace it with the second cloth, keeping your face warm and your body relaxed.

Yields 2 cups

2 cups dried mullein
    leaves, shredded
2 cups water
2 clean cotton cloths

Calendula Facial Astringent

For oily skin, use this toning astringent every morning to dry up excess oil and firm up skin tissues.

Place the calendula petals in a 1-pint glass jar, and cover them with the witch hazel and optional glycerin. Cap the jar, label it, and steep in a dark cabinet for two weeks. Strain the liquid well through cheesecloth and pour it into a clean bottle. Apply it to your face with a cotton ball, rinse lightly, and follow with a light moisturizing cream as desired.

Yields 2 cups

2 cups tightly packed fresh
    calendula petals
2 cups witch hazel
1 teaspoon vegetable
    glycerin (optional)

❧ Acne Internal Tincture

Yields 2 cups

1 cup burdock root,
  cleaned and chopped
1 cup burdock seeds (burs)
1 cup apple cider vinegar
1 cup water

Teenage hormonal changes are completely normal and usually need no herbal or medical interference. However, burdock root and seeds have traditionally been used to alleviate problems directly related to the acne some teens experience during their hormone fluctuations.

Follow the instructions in chapter 4: Medicine-Making Methods for making a vinegar tincture. Take ½ teaspoon 3 times daily in water.

❧ Acne Hormone Balancer

Yields 1 quart

3 tablespoons dried chaste
  tree berry seeds
2 tablespoons dried red
  clover blossoms

Teenage girls often benefit from the use of chaste tree berry, especially when their menstrual cycles are just beginning. Acne can be the result of hormones not yet stabilizing, and this balancing tea can help.

Combine the herbs in a 1-quart glass jar. Pour enough boiling water over them to fill the jar. Follow the instructions in chapter 4: Medicine Making Methods for making an herbal infusion. Drink 2 to 3 cups daily.

HAIR CARE

Your hair says a lot about your health. We'd all like to have shiny, healthy, bouncy, and tangle-free tresses. Symbolic of vitality and indicative of good hygiene, healthy hair is easy to achieve with the following simple herbal preparations (and, of course, a good diet, fresh water, and bountiful sleep). Make fresh batches of these hair care remedies regularly and enjoy them often.

Nettle-Rosemary Hair Rinse for Dark Hair

Lavish your dark locks with this surprisingly rich rinse. Vinegar cleans, strips away old layers of gunk and grime, and leaves hair silky and shiny. Nettles and rosemary add dark depth to the hair and nourish the scalp. Keep this rinse in the refrigerator in the summertime, and use it in the outdoor shower for a cooling rinse. Warm it in the winter before using.

Combine the herbs in a 1-pint glass jar. Warm the vinegar in a pan and pour it over the herbs. Allow it to steep overnight. Strain and reserve the liquid; add the vegetable glycerin. Shake the mixture well. Use 2 to 4 teaspoons per shower instead of or after shampoo. Massage it into the scalp well and rinse.

Yields 2 cups

1 cup dried nettle leaves, chopped
1 cup dried rosemary, chopped
2 cups apple cider vinegar
1 teaspoon vegetable glycerin

Herbal Lemon Hair Rinse for Light Hair

This is a cleansing, lightening formula for blond hair. Rinse it out under the shower, or leave it on while you go play in the sunshine; the sun will lighten your hair even more.

Combine all the ingredients in a 1-pint glass jar. Steep overnight. Strain and reserve the liquid; shake it well. Use 2 to 4 teaspoons per shower instead of or after shampoo. Massage it into the scalp well and rinse.

Yields 2 cups

2 cups fresh calendula blossoms or elder flowers
1¼ cups freshly squeezed lemon juice
¼ cup white vinegar

FACIAL CARE

Herbs and flower preparations have been used for centuries for both men's and women's facial care. Since Maria Prophetissa discovered distillation techniques and created what we call the "bain-marie," chemists and boutiques have sold flower waters and essential oils for beauty applications.

These lovely waters were favorites with ladies throughout the Middle Ages and have never lost their popularity.

With facial care, we generally consider two applications: drying (toning) and moisturizing. Determine your skin type and use whichever remedy will achieve the effect you need. Scent them as desired (lavender is a traditional and lovely facial scent), and enjoy.

Lavender Facial Wash

Yields approximately 1 cup

½ cup fresh lavender flowers
¼ cup rolled oats
1 cup distilled witch hazel
1 teaspoon vegetable
   glycerin
2 to 3 drops lavender
   essential oil

This is a simple-to-make facial astringent that soothes, tightens, and tones the skin. Follow it with Red Clover Whipped Lotion (the recipe follows) for a rich moisturizer.

Combine the dry ingredients and the witch hazel in a 1-pint glass jar; steep overnight or up to two weeks. Strain and reserve the liquid; add the glycerin and essential oil. Using a cotton ball, dab the facial wash over your face using upward motions. (After straining the liquid out, try gently scrubbing your face with the flowers and oats instead of throwing them out; they will remove dirt and grime from the crevasses of your skin and exfoliate. Follow with the facial wash. Delightful!)

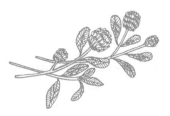

Red Clover Whipped Lotion

Make a tiny batch of this lotion at a time, perhaps for special occasions when you want your face to glow. It's extremely rich and, depending on how much water you add, can be dense or light as a cloud.

Place the herbs and cocoa butter in a bowl. Without heating, use a spoon to mix the blossoms into the cocoa butter. Cover and store in a dark cabinet or pantry. Steep for two weeks.

In the top of a double boiler, gently heat the cocoa butter just until you can strain out the blossoms. Discard them and pour the melted cocoa butter into a deep soup pot (this is to reduce splattering). Using a wire whisk or an electric hand mixer, slowly add the distilled water by the tablespoonful, whisking constantly, until you have the desired consistency. Add the oil if desired, and whisk together. Scrape the lotion into a small container. This lotion lasts several weeks when refrigerated.

Yields 2 to 3 cups

1 cup fresh red clover
blossoms
1 cup cocoa butter
1 to 2 cups distilled water
or rose water
1 to 2 teaspoons jojoba
or sweet almond oil
(optional)

Rose Petal Facial Toner

This is a simple and delightful astringent for the face.

Combine all the ingredients in a 1-pint glass jar. Steep overnight or up to two weeks. Strain and reserve the liquid. If desired, dilute it with additional distilled water or rose water, or whisk in a few drops of vegetable glycerin. Apply this toner with a cotton ball, using upward strokes.

Yields 2 cups

1 cup packed fresh rose
petals
1 cup distilled witch hazel
1 cup distilled water
Rose water or vegetable
glycerin (optional)

Dandelion-Elder Flower Blemish Lightener

Yields 2 cups

1 cup fresh elder flowers
1 cup fresh dandelion
    flowers
2 cups fresh buttermilk

*Adapted from old wives' recipes, this classic blemish lightener uses butter-
milk. Many old recipes call for tansy flowers, but I find elder flower to be just
as lovely.*

Combine all the ingredients in a glass jar. Steep overnight in the refrigerator (refrigeration is important!). Strain and reserve the liquid. Using a cotton ball, apply the lotion to your face in upward movements. Once your
face is covered, lie down and rest for 10 minutes. Rinse with cool water.
Store this lotion in the refrigerator for up to two weeks.

Lemon Lip Balm

Yields 1 cup

1 cup fresh lemon balm (or
    herb of your choice),
    chopped
1 cup vegetable oil (such as
    canola)
¼ cup beeswax
2 to 5 drops lemon
    essential oil or high-
    quality culinary lemon
    extract

*Lemon is a luscious, summery fragrance, and many of our beloved herbs offer
that scent: lemon balm, lemon verbena, lemongrass, and wood sorrel (Oxalis)
leaves and seedpods. Pick your favorites to infuse in the oil for this lip balm.*

Follow the instructions in chapter 4: Medicine-Making Methods for making an herbal salve. Once the wax has melted, pour the mixture into small
lip balm tubes or into ¼-ounce tins. Because these small containers absorb
heat easily, do not keep them in pants pockets or in a hot car.

BODY CARE

Massages and deep, relaxing baths are special forms of body care. Not generally considered medicinal, they are nevertheless soothing and healing.
Aromatherapy plays a large part in these wonderful remedies; it is the sci-

ence of scent and its ability to transform our state of mind (and therefore the physical body) simply with fragrance.

The oils in this section can be used directly on the skin, in the hair, on the feet, or in the bath, being sure to avoid the eyes. Be lavish with the scent in these products, which will stay fragrant two to three years when capped tightly and stored in a dark cabinet.

Lavender Massage and Body Oil

This rich massage oil is strongly scented with lavender and makes a wonderful body or bath oil. It penetrates quickly and leaves a silky feel to the skin. We sell out quickly in early summer.

Combine the flowers and grapeseed oil in a glass jar; steep for two weeks in a dark place. Strain and reserve the oil. With a wire whisk, blend in the essential oil and the contents of the vitamin E capsule, if using. Store the oil in plastic or glass bottles with tight-fitting lids. Enjoy!

Yields 2 cups

1 cup fresh lavender flowers
2 cups grapeseed oil,
    sweet almond oil, jojoba
    oil, hempseed oil, and/
    or macadamia nut oil
10 to 20 drops lavender
    essential oil
Vitamin E capsule
    (optional)

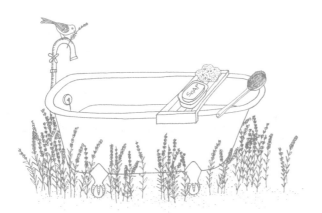

Sensual Massage and Body Oil

30 drops of the following in any combination: amyris (*Amyris balsamifera*) essential oil, Peru balsam (*Myroxylon balsamum*) essential oil, and nutmeg essential oil

5 drops pure vanilla extract

2 cups grapeseed oil, sweet almond oil, jojoba oil, hempseed oil, and/or macadamia nut oil

Vitamin E capsule (optional)

A decadent and exotic scent, the essential oils in this preparation combine to create a truly mesmerizing massage, body, or bath oil. These scents mimic sandalwood, a valuable plant that is overharvested; using these herbs gives the same quality without endangering a threatened plant supply. The oils can be found at high-quality health food stores or from suppliers in the Resource section at the back of this book.

Combine all the ingredients in a bowl. Break open the capsule and add the vitamin E, if using, and whisk together. Pour the oil into plastic or glass bottles with tight-fitting lids. Shake well before using.

Lavender Flower Water Body Spritzer

Yields 1 cup

½ cup witch hazel

½ cup water

10 to 20 drops lavender essential oil (or scent of your choice)

Nothing is more refreshing on a hot summer day than spritzing your face, neck, body, and even pillow and linens with cool lavender flower water. A true hydrosol is steam-distilled using special machinery, but since most people don't have access to distillers, this recipe uses lavender essential oil, which is available at most health food stores. Feel free to substitute other scents; sweet orange is a lovely summer scent with refreshing, awakening qualities.

Combine all the ingredients in a spray bottle. Kept in the fridge, this makes a lovely summer spray. *Note:* Some recipes include vegetable glycerin, but I don't recommend using it in these sprays, as it can stain linens.

Chapter Eighteen

HERBAL DRINKS, DRESSINGS, AND OTHER EDIBLES

The Greek philosopher and healer Hippocrates said, "If we could give every individual the right amount of nourishment and exercise, not too little and not too much, we would have found the safest way to health." Even today, this is valid advice. The nourishing foods we consume are the foundation of our health, and they affect us as much (or more so) than the medications and even herbal remedies we consume.

The recipes presented here are for fun things you can make in your kitchen, whether warming spirits, cordials, and liqueurs, or main dishes for dinner. Often you can get a lot of nutrition out of these foods and beverages, though they are not formatted for doses—only enjoyment.

CORDIALS

If you enjoy making tinctures, you'll want to experiment with cordials. A cordial is a liqueur—a sweet, sometimes floral, sometimes fruity alcoholic drink. It comes in as wide a range of flavors as all the berries and flowers you can find, but they all generally have the same mouthfeel: a smooth, velvety texture that is luscious and creamy. Often cordials contain cream or chocolate syrup, but you can make them strictly with berries or even nuts and get the same deliciousness without the extra calories. They make wonderful gifts, and a little goes a long way. Stock up on one- and two-quart glass jars, and be prepared to make them long in advance; if you want to give Hanukkah or Christmas gifts, begin making your cordials in summer and early autumn with fresh fruit and flowers.

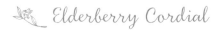 Elderberry Cordial

Yields approximately 1 quart

2 quarts fresh elderberries

1 cup sugar

2 cups vodka

1 cup brandy

2 tablespoons lemon juice

This is one of my favorites. Elderberries are among my favorite trees for their medicine, and I use every bit of them: berries, leaves, flowers, and twigs. Here, the berries make a divine liqueur with a gorgeous purple color that needs to be shown off in a clear glass decanter. This recipe produces a lightly sweet, lightly tart, fruity cordial with a silky mouthfeel.

In a glass 2-quart jar, crush the elderberries with a long-handled wooden spoon. Pour in the sugar and crush them together, being sure to appreciate the amazing scarlet color! (Wear appropriate clothing or an apron, as elderberry juice will stain fabrics blue.) Pour in the vodka, brandy, and lemon juice; and cover the mixture with water or more vodka until it is ¼ inch from the top of the jar. Cap the jar and shake it; label and store it in a cool, dark place for at least two months. Decant (strain) the mixture into a clean jar, and discard the berry matter. Test the flavor for sweetness, but realize that it will mellow over time. Store for one more month, and decant the liqueur again through cheesecloth if desired.

Rose Brandy

Pick the most fragrant rose petals you can find; often the wild roses (Rosa rugosa) that grow along Martha's Vineyard's Aquinnah and Oak Bluffs beaches are beautiful but not too fragrant. Find flowers that smell heavenly but have not been sprayed with any pesticides or herbicides.

Gather enough rose petals to fill a 1-quart glass jar. Don't chop the petals; instead, press them tightly into the jar. Make sugar syrup: In a saucepan, heat the water and sugar until clear, stirring constantly. Allow to cool. Pour this syrup and the brandy over the petals. Cap and label the jar. Steep for two months in a cool, dark place. Strain the liquid; add drops of vanilla to taste. Pour into a clean bottle and return to the cool, dark place and allow it to age at least one more month.

Serve this brandy at room temperature or chilled, or drizzle it over vanilla ice cream or lemon cake.

Yields approximately 3 cups

1 quart fresh rose petals, packed (5 to 6 cups)
1 cup water
1 cup sugar
2 cups brandy
Vanilla extract

Hazelnut Liqueur

This liqueur makes an intensely sweet sipping drink with the heavenly aroma of hazelnuts. Hazelnuts (filberts) grow wild on Martha's Vineyard; occasionally my family treks out to collect them, but we are often beaten to the punch by raccoons and squirrels, and those nuts we do collect turn out to be tiny. If you can harvest fresh nuts, all the better, though store-bought nuts make a good product too.

Place the nuts in a 1-quart jar, and pour the vodka and brandy over them. Make sugar syrup: In a saucepan, heat the water and sugar until clear, stirring constantly. Allow to cool. Pour this into the jar, and top off with more vodka until the liquid reaches ¼ inch of the top of the jar. Cap the jar, label

Yields 2 to 3 cups

2 cups hazelnuts, chopped
1 cup vodka
1 cup brandy
½ cup water
½ cup sugar
Vanilla or hazelnut extract

it, and steep for two months. Strain the liquid; add vanilla or hazelnut extract to taste. Pour into a clean bottle and allow the liqueur to age one more month. *Note:* The hazelnuts absorb quite a bit of liquid, so the resulting liqueur amount is not as much as with berry liqueurs. After straining, you can add the spiked nuts to baking recipes instead of composting them.

🌿 *Hot "Love Liqueur" with Cardamom*

Yields 2 cups

1 cup fresh rose hips, chopped

1 cup fresh elderberries or black cherries

¼ cup dried hibiscus

¼ cup dried cardamom seeds, crushed

2 star anise

1 tablespoon orange zest

4 to 5 whole cloves

1 cup vodka

½ cup rum or brandy

½ cup water

½ cup sugar

2 tablespoons honey

Sweet orange extract (optional)

A spicy, fruity cordial, this is wonderful slightly heated and drizzled over vanilla ice cream or cherry cobbler. Or heat it and serve in a small liqueur glass with a few drops of fresh cream. Divine!

Fill a 1-quart glass jar with the berries and spices. Pour the vodka and rum over them. Make sugar syrup: In a saucepan, heat the water and sugar until clear, stirring constantly. Stir in the honey. Allow to cool slightly. Pour this syrup into the jar and top it off with more rum or water until the liquid reaches ¼ inch of the top of the jar. Cap the jar and label it. Steep for two months. Strain the liquid; add the sweet orange extract if desired. Pour into a clean bottle and allow the liqueur to age another month before serving.

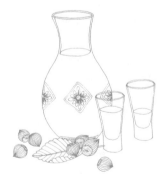

Autumn Olive Smooth Liqueur

What a delicious cordial! Autumn olives are of the Elaeagnus genus and are considered an invasive species; here on Martha's Vineyard, they are considered a pest, and there might even be a law against planting them. But the berries are tart and tasty, and the U.S. Department of Agriculture notes that they are high in lycopene (and probably antioxidants). The berries make tart fruit leather and, combined with blueberries, a delicious pie, but by far their best use is in a liqueur. With time (after a year or so), this liqueur turns from tart and tangy to the smoothest, mellowest, and richest alcoholic beverage you will ever try.

Yields approximately 1 quart

2 quarts fresh autumn
    olive berries, pits and all
2 cups vodka
1 cup brandy or rum
1 cup water
1 cup sugar
Flavoring extract of choice
    (I prefer almond or
    vanilla)

Fill a 2-quart glass jar with the berries and crush them with a long-handled wooden spoon. Pour in the vodka and brandy. Make sugar syrup: In a saucepan, heat the water and sugar until clear, stirring constantly. Allow to cool slightly. Pour this syrup into the jar and top it off with more vodka or water until the liquid reaches ¼ inch of the top of the jar. Cap the jar, label it, and steep for two months. Strain the liquid; add the flavoring extract to taste. Pour into a clean bottle and allow to age at least another month.

SALAD DRESSINGS

Getting your daily herbs can be tasty. These salad dressings make wonderful additions to the family dinner table and, as my son can attest, make salads the most desirable part of the meal. He loves vinegar, and the Dandelion Dandy Salad Dressing is a tart favorite—plus it's naturally high in iron and potassium. Make it during the summer to keep on hand year-round; it keeps well, especially if you add the oil just before serving.

For Easy Salad Vinegar, Delicious Spring Salad, and Spring Asparagus Meal, refer to chapter 15: Cleansing and Detox. For Iron-Rich Salad Dressing, refer to chapter 7: Especially for Women.

Dandelion Dandy Salad Vinegar

Yields 2 cups

2 cups fresh dandelion
    root, chopped
1 cup fresh dandelion
    leaves, chopped
2 cups apple cider vinegar

Used alone, this vinegar is flavorful and rich in iron; it is also the basis for the Dandelion Dandy Salad Dressing (recipe follows).

Wash the dandelion roots and chop them along with the leaves. In a saucepan, heat the vinegar to a simmer. Place the roots and leaves in a 1-quart glass jar and pour the warm vinegar over them. Cap the jar, label it, and store it in a cool, dark cabinet for two weeks, placing the jar on a plate in case of leakage. Strain the vinegar and return the liquid to a clean jar. Label and store in a cabinet.

Dandelion Dandy Salad Dressing

Yields 2 cups

½ cup Dandelion Dandy
    Salad Vinegar
¼ teaspoon honey
1½ cups olive oil
Spices and herbs of
    your choice, such as
    fresh or dried parsley,
    Mexican oregano, and
    granulated garlic
Salt and pepper

This dressing combines the vinegar (see above) with olive oil for delicious salads.

In a medium-sized bowl, whisk together honey and oil. Add the vinegar to the oil and whisk in the herbs, salt, and pepper to taste. Store the dressing in a glass jar in the pantry.

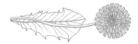

Sweet Wildflower Zinger Salad Vinegar

This flavorful vinegar allows you to revel in those beautiful summer colors before they fade. Harvest a mountain of wildflowers and preserve them in this vinegar dressing; it's not too tart and lets the delicate flavors of the wildflowers shine through. By making the vinegar separately from the oil, you can use what you need when you're ready to serve a salad and save the remaining vinegar for another time (see the Sweet Wildflower Zinger Salad Dressing recipe below). Drizzle this vinegar on fresh, buttery lettuce leaves; fresh vegetables; and even certain fruits, like pears and peaches, served with thinly sliced sharp cheeses.

Roughly chop the wildflowers and leaves. In a saucepan, heat the vinegar to a simmer. Place the wildflowers and leaves in a 1-quart glass jar and pour the warm vinegar over them. Cap the jar, label it, and store it in a cool, dark cabinet for two weeks, placing the jar on a plate in case of leakage. Strain the vinegar and return the liquid to a clean jar. Label and store in a cabinet.

Yields 2 cups

3 cups packed fresh
   wildflowers and leaves
   (red clover, lemon
   balm, mint, nasturtium,
   wood sorrel, Saint-
   John's-wort, violets,
   elder flowers, and so
   on)
2 cups white wine vinegar
   or light balsamic vinegar

Sweet Wildflower Zinger Salad Dressing

This dressing combines the vinegar (see above) with olive oil for delicious salads.

In a medium-sized bowl, whisk together honey and oil. Add the vinegar to the oil and whisk in the herbs, salt, and pepper to taste. Store the dressing in a glass jar in the pantry.

Yields 2 cups

½ cup Sweet Wildflower
   Zinger Salad Vinegar
¼ teaspoon honey
1½ cups olive oil
Spices and herbs of
   your choice, such
   as granulated garlic,
   lovage, rosemary, stevia,
   and so on
Salt and pepper

DELICIOUS SYRUPS

Herbal syrups are easy and quick to prepare, and they make a lovely addition to teas. I often stir a teaspoon of elder flower or mint syrup into my hot herbal teas in the winter instead of sugar or plain honey. The flavor is delicate, enticing, and floral, and it always reminds me of who was with me when I harvested a particular plant. Store these syrups in the fridge and expect them to last two to four months—unless you use them up beforehand!

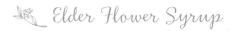 Elder Flower Syrup

Yields approximately 1 cup

1 cup water

1 cup packed fresh elder flowers

½ cup sweetener (honey, granulated sugar, turbinado, and so on)

My talented friend Kirstin Uhrenholdt, a private chef and coauthor of A Family Dinner with Laurie David and others, shared with me her elder flower syrup woes when her batch turned gooey. I've experienced it too: the liquidy texture of the syrup changes from smooth and pourable to snotlike and unappetizing. "Danish lore warns us to ask permission from the Elderberry witch before picking her flowers," Kirstin says, "and I think the reason my syrup became possessed was that my request was not granted." In addition to asking permission and refrigerating the finished syrup, I believe the answer lies in the length of time you steep the flowers. Take care not to steep them in the hot water too long. A quick dunk is sufficient to capture the tantalizing flavor and scent of elder flowers while keeping a clean, liquidy syrup. This varies from my method of making other syrups, which requires a long steeping period that allows most of the water to evaporate. Note: The choice of sweetener is up to you, but I've had the best results with plain granulated sugar or honey.

In a saucepan, bring the water to a boil. Plunge the elder flowers into the hot water and let them steep, covered, for only 5 to 7 minutes. Strain the mixture, pouring the liquid back into the saucepan. Add the sweetener, and stir over low heat just until blended. Pour the syrup into a 1-pint jar and store it in the refrigerator.

Elderberry Pancake Syrup

What to do with all those plump, purple elderberries? Originally published in Martha's Vineyard Magazine, *this tasty pancake and waffle syrup is one of my family's favorites for enjoying on a cold winter morning.*

In a large soup pot, boil the elderberries with the water (uncovered) for 1 hour, or until the water is reduced by about half. This makes a strong, rich tea. Strain the tea.

Pour the tea back into the soup pot and add the sugar. Bring to a boil, then simmer, stirring frequently, until the sugar dissolves and the tea thickens, about 15 minutes.

Remove from the heat and allow to cool. Add the maple syrup. Bottle in clear jars to show off the gorgeous color, and serve warm over pancakes, waffles, oatmeal, granola, and fresh fruit. This recipe yields enough to keep some for yourself and give the rest as gifts.

Yields 4 to 5 cups

½ gallon fresh or frozen elderberries (some stem is fine)

2 quarts fresh water

3 cups sugar (or less, to taste)

3 to 4 tablespoons maple syrup

Peppermint-Ginger Pancake Syrup

This is a sweet syrup with a little zing. It's wonderful as a sweetener for West Chop Winter Tea for Colds and Flu *(see chapter 10: Sniffles, Colds, and Viruses) or as a treat for someone who needs a pick-me-up. Warming, stimulating, and fragrant.*

In a large saucepan, combine the peppermint, ginger, and water. Bring to a boil, then lower the heat and simmer until the volume has decreased to approximately 1 cup. This creates a strong, fragrant tea. Strain the liquid and return it to the pot. Add the sweetener, and heat gently until completely blended. Store the syrup in a 1-pint jar in the refrigerator.

Yields about 3 cups

½ cup fresh peppermint leaves, chopped

½ cup fresh ginger, chopped (skin is fine)

3 cups water

½ cup sweetener (honey or sugar)

Rose Petal Tea Syrup

Yields about 1 cup

3 cups fresh rose petals
3 cups water
½ cup honey

By far, this is the most delectable tea sweetener. Use a teaspoon of this lovely syrup in your hot tea, or sweeten cold lemon tea with it.

In a large saucepan, combine the petals and water. Bring to a boil, then lower the heat and simmer until the volume has decreased to approximately 1 cup. Strain the liquid and return it to the pot. Add the honey, and gently heat until the mixture is completely blended. Store the syrup in a 1-pint jar in the refrigerator.

HERBAL HONEYS

Honeys are different from syrups in that the herb is infused directly into the raw honey; there is no infusion to make first. These are among the easiest recipes involving herbs and absolutely the most enjoyable to consume. The honeys retain their nutrients and enzymes because they are subjected to a minimum of heat, and the flavor is spectacular. Use mild honeys, such as clover, to allow the herb's flavor to shine through. Each recipe makes six 8-ounce jars to give as gifts, with a homemade label indicating the honey is delicious on toast and muffins and in tea.

Lavender Honey

Yields 4 to 6 cups

5 to 6 cups fresh lavender
    flowers, chopped
48 ounces (1 large can)
    honey
1 drop lavender essential
    oil (optional)

Lavender blossoms infuse this honey with a summer scent that's wonderful on biscuits. Use the strongest-scented lavender you can find.

Place the flowers in a soup pot. Pour the honey over them, poking with a long-handled wooden spoon to ensure that all the flowers are covered. Allow this mixture to sit overnight, or even up to three nights, covered with a lid.

Place the pot on very low heat. When the honey turns to a liquid (just a few minutes), immediately strain into jars. Press the herbs to release every bit of the honey, and compost the herbs. Add the essential oil, if using, and stir. Cap the jars and store them in a cabinet.

Wild Mint Honey

Refreshing and eye-opening, this honey is a delicious reminder of summer throughout the winter. Stir it into hot teas or into a morning bowl of oatmeal.

Yields 4 to 6 cups

5 to 6 cups fresh mint leaves, chopped

48 ounces (1 large can) honey

Place the mint leaves in a soup pot. Pour the honey over them, poking with a long-handled wooden spoon to ensure that all the leaves are covered with honey. Allow this mixture to sit overnight, or even up to three nights, covered with a lid.

Place the pot on low heat. When the honey turns to a liquid (just a few minutes), immediately strain it into jars. Press the herbs to release every bit of the honey, and compost the herbs. This honey is fragrant; no essential oil is needed. Cap the jars and store them in a cabinet.

DIVINE BEVERAGES

Chilled or hot, sweetened or not, herbs make wonderful drinks. Here are several ways to enjoy them.

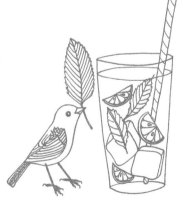

Iced Lemon Tisane

Yields 3 to 4 cups

3 cups water

1 cup packed fresh lemon
  balm leaves, chopped

½ cup fresh lemon juice

2 stevia leaves or 1
  teaspoon Rose Petal Tea
  Syrup (see the "Delicious
  Syrups" section)

This mild, lemony drink is lightly sweet and ideal for "tea and biscuits" on the back porch. The lemon balm leaves add a refreshing herbal taste to the familiar lemon zing.

Bring the water to a boil. Place the lemon balm leaves in a kettle. Pour the hot water over the leaves and cover; steep for 8 to 10 minutes. Strain. To the liquid, add lemon juice and stevia or syrup. Steep for 2 more minutes before serving hot, or pour the tisane into a jar and refrigerate it for iced tea. Garnish with a sprig of lemon balm or stevia.

Summer Herb and Black Tea

Black tea (Camellia sinensis) blends deliciously with citrus. My Edgartown English Breakfast tea is a blend of broken orange pekoe black teas and chopped orange peel, and the flavors balance each other perfectly. Make this tea hot or cold; it's best sweetened with granulated sugar.

To Make One Cup

1 cup water

1 teaspoon black tea
  (English breakfast, Irish
  breakfast, etc.)

3 teaspoons dried lemon
  balm leaves (or 1 small
  handful fresh)

½ teaspoon dried lemon or
  orange peel

¼ teaspoon sugar

Bring the water to a boil. Place the black tea, lemon balm leaves, and dried lemon or orange peel in a kettle, and pour the water over them. Steep for 5 to 7 minutes, or to desired strength. Strain the tea, and add the sugar. Serve immediately for hot tea, or refrigerate for cold.

To Make A Pitcher

In a large pot, bring the water to a boil. Add the tea, herbs, citrus peel, and sugar to the pot; remove from the heat and cover. Steep for 10 minutes, then strain and let the tea cool. Refrigerate it at least 3 hours before serving.

8 cups water

1 cup black tea (or 8 tea bags)

2 cups fresh lemon balm leaves, chopped

¼ cup dried lemon or orange peel

¾ to 1 cup sugar

Rich Winter Herbal Hot Cocoa

Nothing beats hot chocolate in the winter, but if you'd like to try an equally wonderful, silky, and nourishing hot drink, indulge in a mug of this dandelion-cocoa. Don't skimp on the sugar, since both cocoa and dandelion are naturally bitter. (For suppliers of ready-made dandelion drinks, see the Resources section at the back of this book.)

Put the cocoa powder, dandelion root, cinnamon, and sugar in a kettle. Pour the water over them and stir well. When blended, add the heavy cream and divide into four mugs.

Yields 4 to 5 cups

2 tablespoons cocoa powder

1 tablespoon powdered dandelion root or powdered chicory root

½ teaspoon powdered cinnamon

2 to 3 tablespoons sugar

4 cups boiling water

½ cup heavy cream

✾ Summer Mint Ice Cubes

Yields about 1½ trays

3 cups small leaves
  or flowers (such as
  peppermint, spearmint,
  lemon balm, or apple
  mint), divided

2 cups boiling water

Almost any herb or flower can go into these lovely ice cubes to grace a summer glass of water, lemonade, tea, or punch. Part of your harvest goes into the flavoring, and part is reserved for "looks."

Place 2 cups of the herbs into a kettle or pot, and pour the water over them. Steep, covered, for 8 to 10 minutes. Strain the liquid and return it to the pot. Cover and allow it to cool. Pour the tea into ice cube trays and place them in the freezer. After about 20 minutes, pull the trays out; as they begin to freeze, insert one fresh leaf or flower into each cube. (*Note:* If the leaves are large, curl them into the tray first, before you pour the tea in.) Return the trays to the freezer. Serve the ice cubes in individual glasses for cold drinks, or plunge many cubes into a large glass pitcher of your favorite beverage.

Dosage Guidelines

Determining the proper dose for an herbal remedy is as much subjective as it is objective. Even over-the-counter medicines must offer a range of doses on their labels because every person varies by weight, constitution, and even allergic response. Standard doses simply cannot be given for any medicine to address every person during every illness. For this reason, intuition is useful, as is an understanding of the general properties of the herbs. Dosages vary, too, based on the herb used as well as the illness. Use common sense and always start with the smallest dose and work up as needed.

I've found that so-called standard herbal doses are generally intended for men or heavier women; Clark's rule, a formula for calculating doses, implies that a standard adult dose is appropriate for a 150-pound person. If you're slender and light, or if you're heavier than 150 pounds, this rule is not ideal for you. Other herbal dosage rules (such as Cowling's and Young's) have you computing, measuring, and dividing—all based on age. This is nonsense, as people's weights vary widely even when they are the same age.

A weight-based dose is most appropriate. In general, when medicating children, divide an adult dose by three—or better yet, consider the weight of the child in comparison to the weight of an adult. A 60-pound child needs only one-third to one-half the dose for a 150-pound adult. (*Note:* The guidelines provided here are only suggestions based on experience and herbal tradition; they are not meant to take the place of the advice of a qualified health practitioner.)

The following guidelines are divided into sections. First are the adult doses for acute and chronic conditions. Second are the children's doses, which are further divided by weight. For example, if you are dosing a 66-pound boy with echinacea root decoction for a sinus infection, look under "Children," "Acute Condition," his weight, and then "Tea." At the end of the guidelines, you'll find recommendations for infant doses.

Tea refers to teas, infusions, and decoctions. *Tincture* refers to tinctures, syrups, and concentrates.

ADULTS

Acute condition

Tea: 1 cup every hour (for a total of 4 cups per day)
Tincture: 1 teaspoon every hour

Chronic condition

Tea: 3 to 4 cups daily
Tincture: 1 teaspoon 3 times daily

Illness prevention and nourishment

Tea: 2 to 3 cups daily
Tincture: ½ teaspoon 2 to 3 times daily

CHILDREN

Acute condition

15–45 pounds (ages 2 to 6):
Tea: ¼ cup every hour (for a total of 1 cup per day)
Tincture: 10 drops (⅛ teaspoon) every hour

46–75 pounds (ages 7 to 11):
    Tea: ¹/₃ cup every hour (for a total of 1¹/₃ cups per day)
    Tincture: 20 drops (¼ teaspoon) every hour
76–125 pounds (ages 12 to 18):
    Tea: ½ cup every hour (for a total of 2 cups per day)
    Tincture: 40 drops (½ teaspoon) every hour

Chronic condition

15–45 pounds (ages 2 to 6): Tea: ¼ cup 3 times daily
    Tincture: 10 drops (¹/₈ teaspoon) 3 times daily
46–75 pounds (ages 7 to 11): Tea: ¹/₃ cup 3 times daily
    Tincture: 20 drops (¼ teaspoon) 3 times daily
76–125 pounds (ages 12 to 18): Tea: ½ cup 3 times daily
    Tincture: 40 drops (½ teaspoon) 3 times daily

Illness Prevention and Nourishment

Most preventive and nourishing herbal teas and infusions are safe in whatever amount a child will take, since children will generally drink only what
feels best to them. Start with small, unsweetened amounts such as ¼ cup,
served in a teacup or mug, and allow your child to drink as much red clover, nettle, alfalfa, lemon balm, and other nutritive teas as she wishes. Keep
dandelion (a diuretic) and licorice brews to a minimum. Nettle teas, while
nourishing, sometimes cause diarrhea. If this happens, simply dilute the tea
with water or alternate cups of water with cups of tea.

Teas are the best form of medicine for preventing illness and nourishing
your child's body, though syrups are acceptable (halve the chronic condition
dose). Tinctures generally are not appropriate.

For Nursing Infants

Infants receive the best medicine through their mother's breast milk, so the
mother usually drinks the medicine (this won't work when the baby needs

astringent herbs to address diarrhea or runny sinuses, since the herbs will dry up the breast milk). Some mothers like to dip their finger in a cup of tea for the baby to suck, or they'll place a dropper beside their nipple while the baby is nursing so 2 to 3 drops of tincture can be given. Also, 2 to 3 drops of tincture or ½ teaspoon of plain herbal tea can be added directly to formula in the bottle. Because honey can contain botulism spores, never give honey herbal preparations to infants younger than one year.

DROPS IN A TEASPOON

Various sources report the number of drops in a teaspoon differently. Measure for yourself. Here's my formula:

20 drops = ¼ teaspoon
80 to 90 drops = 1 teaspoon

Seasonal Chart for Harvesting Herbs

Calendula   Summer, fall
Catnip   Spring, summer, fall
Dandelion flowers   Summer, fall
Dandelion leaves   Spring, summer, fall,
    early winter
Dandelion root   Fall, early winter
Elder flowers   Summer
Elder leaves   Fall
Elderberries   Fall
Ginger   Purchase anytime
Lavender   Summer
Lemon balm   Summer
Marshmallow root   Summer, fall
Mints   Spring, summer, fall,
    early winter

Motherwort   Summer
Mullein   Summer, fall
Nettle   Spring
Plantain   Summer, fall
Red clover   Summer, fall
Rose hips   Fall
Rose petals   Summer
Violet flowers   Spring
Violet leaves   Spring, summer
Wild sarsaparilla   Fall
Yarrow flowers   Summer
Yarrow leaves   Summer, fall, early
    winter

Common Plant Names and Their Latin Binomials

Here is a list of the common names of all the Essential Herbs, plus additional herbs mentioned in this book. Since several herbs can share the same common name, making certain identification questionable, the Latin binomials (or "official" names) help guarantee we are talking about the same plant.

Angelica   *Angelica archangelica*
Arnica   *Arnica montana*
Ashwagandha   *Withania somnifera*
Astragalus   *Astragalus membranaceus*
Autumn olive   *Elaeagnus umbellata*
Blessed thistle   *Cnicus benedictus*
Boneset   *Eupatorium perfoliatum*
Borage   *Borago officinalis*
Burdock   *Arctium lappa*
Calendula   *Calendula officinalis*
Catnip   *Nepeta cataria*
Cayenne   *Capsicum minimum*
Chamomile   *Matricaria recutita*
Chaste tree berry   *Vitex agnus-castus*
Chicory   *Cichorium intybus*
Crampbark   *Viburnum opulus*
Cranesbill   *Geranium maculatum*
Damiana   *Turnera diffusa*
Dandelion   *Taraxacum officinale*
Dill   *Anethum graveolens*
Echinacea   *Echinacea angustifolia, E. purpurea*
Elder   *Sambucus nigra, S. canadensis*

Evening primrose   *Oenothera biennis*
Fennel   *Foeniculum vulgare*
Fenugreek   *Trigonella foenum-graecum*
Feverfew   *Tanacetum parthenium*
Fo-ti   *Polygonum multiflorum*
Garlic   *Allium sativum*
Ginger   *Zingiber officinale*
Ginseng   *Panax* spp.
Goldenseal   *Hydrastis canadensis*
Hawthorn   *Crataegus oxyacanthoides*
Hazelnut   *Corylus americana*
Hops   *Humulus lupulus*
Jewelweed   *Impatiens* spp.
Lady's mantle   *Alchemilla mollis*
Lavender   *Lavandula officinalis, L. angustifolia*
Lemon balm   *Melissa officinalis*
Linden   *Tilia* spp.
Marshmallow   *Althaea officinalis*
Milk thistle   *Silybum marianum*
Motherwort   *Leonurus cardiaca*
Mugwort   *Artemisia vulgaris*
Mullein   *Verbascum thapsus*

Nettle   *Urtica dioica*
Oatstraw   *Avena sativa*
Passionflower   *Passiflora incarnata*
Peppermint   *Mentha piperita*
Plantain   *Plantago major, P. lanceolata*
Prickly ash   *Zanthoxylum americanum*
Raspberry   *Rubus idaeus, R. strigosus*
Red clover   *Trifolium pratense*
Rose   *Rosa* spp.
Sage   *Salvia officinalis*
Saint-John's-wort   *Hypericum perforatum*
Sarsaparilla   *Smilax* spp.
Sassafras   *Sassafras albidum*
Skullcap   *Scutellaria lateriflora*
Slippery elm   *Ulmus rubra* (formerly *Ulmus fulva*)

Spearmint   *Mentha spicata*
Spilanthes   *Spilanthes oleracea, Acmella oleracea*
Thyme   *Thymus* spp.
Valerian   *Valeriana officinalis*
Vervain   *Verbena officinalis*
Violet   *Viola odorata, V. tricolor*
White Willow   *Salix alba*
Wild cherry   *Prunus avium*
Wild lettuce   *Lactuca virosa*
Wild sarsaparilla   *Aralia nudicaulis*
Wild yam   *Dioscorea villosa*
Witch hazel   *Hamamelis virginiana*
Yarrow   *Achillea millefolium*
Yellow dock   *Rumex crispus*

Glossary

alterative: Altering the way the body reacts to stressful situations, whether environmental, physical, or emotional. Herbs such as red clover help the body maintain calm and normal function in the face of anxiety, stress, or toxins.

anti-: The prefix *anti-* precedes the description of many herbal medicines these days. Antibacterial, antifungal, antiviral, anticoagulant, anti-this, anti-that. Usually, these herbs are strong germ and bacteria fighters that either stimulate the body's immune response or actually kill germs on contact. They are very useful for both internal and external applications. In some cases, these herbs must be used with caution (such as the vermifuge wormwood or the antiparasitic rue). Though it seems a negative way of looking at herbs (rather than using the prefix *pro-*, as in probiotic, prohealth, and so on), this is a useful classification that tells you when to use certain herbs. For instance, knowing lemon balm is both nervine and antiviral indicates that it may be a good choice for treating ulcers.

astringent: Drying. Astringent tonics pull skin together, tightening the pores and improving skin tone. They are also useful on weepy sores or blisters and to heal wounds. Internally, astringents ease bloating and diarrhea.

beeswax: When purchasing beeswax, look for unbleached and unfiltered wax. Many health food stores sell beeswax in the form of little beads or as eight-inch sticks. These are heavily processed and should be used only as a last resort, because they result in sticky salves with a strange, mushy consistency. Ask your retailer to stock or special order unfiltered, unbleached blocks of beeswax from which you can shave or cut pieces. Also, see the Resources section in the back of this book.

compress: The medicinal topical application of a warm, wet herbal infusion via a soft cloth or flannel. Similar to a poultice, but a compress uses the liquids from the herbs instead of the herbs themselves. Compresses are usually applied when hot, but they are sometimes applied cold. *Also called* fomentation.

decant: To strain, or pour off liquid. For example, the cordials in this book are decanted simply through a strainer or sieve. A two-foot length of plastic tubing and suction can also be used to remove all traces of plant matter.

decoction: An herbal beverage in which belowground parts of herbs—such as roots or barks, seeds, and hard berries—are steeped for several hours, then strained.

dedicated: Specifically used for herbal medicine making and not shared with other kitchen duties.

demulcent: A herb that is high in mucilage and soothing to either the digestive tract or the skin. Such herbs include plantain leaf and marshmallow root.

diaphoretic: An herb or remedy that causes perspiration, either through the dilation of surface capillaries or through the raising of body temperature. Often diaphoretics are used during colds and influenza to "break" fevers, or in cases of poor cardiac circulation.

diuretic: An herb or remedy that increases the flow of blood through the kidneys and of fluids through the urinary tract. Diurectics increase the volume of urine excreted and are often employed to rid the body of excess water, relieve water-weight gain, or generally tone and support the urinary tract system.

essential oil: The concentrated volatile oil of a plant, usually obtained through distillation. It takes a great deal of plant matter to extract even a tiny bit of essential oil. Often these oils are extremely fragrant and also antibacterial; as such, they are useful as additions to salves and lotions.

flower essence: The energetic component of a plant. Captured through water collection, flower essences address the spiritual and/or emotional needs of the person who takes them.

fomentation: *See* compress.

hepatic: An herb that stimulates and strengthens the liver during jaundice, hormonal imbalance, toxin cleansing, and so on.

herbal medicine: One of the most ancient forms of healing based on the application of plants, plant extracts, or plant parts, either internally or externally. Most herbal, or botanical, medicines are concentrated extracts of a specific plant (as opposed to homeopathic preparations, which are dilutions). Herbal medicines can be used safely for babies and the elderly, although some preparations (like the plants from which they derive) are toxic and must be used with care. Herbal medicine is versatile, functional, nourishing, specific, and holistic.

homeopathy: Attributed to German scientist Samuel Hahnemann in 1796, homeopathy is the use of diluted herbal, mineral, and animal ingredients for medicine. Unlike herbal medicine, which is concentrated, homeopathy is extremely diluted—so much so that some claim that little if any of the original substance is left in the medicine. Homeopathy assumes that "like treats like"; therefore, if a substance such as arsenic makes you vomit, then the diluted form of arsenic will stop you from vomiting. *See* herbal medicine.

hydrosol: The distilled volatile oils and waters of a plant. A true hydrosol is a fragile thing and usually smells strongly of the plant from which it is processed. Often made of fragrant and pleasant herbs, hydrosols are frequently sprayed on the face and body, and even on clothing and linens. The fragrance is short-lived but refreshing.

infusion: An herbal beverage in which aboveground parts of herbs—such as leaves and flowers—are steeped for several hours, then strained. Generally four hours is the minimum time required for herbs to release their minerals into hot water. For this reason, infusions are considered much more medicinal than tisanes. *See also* decoction.

laxative: An herb that stimulates bowel movements during constipation.

liniment: A concentrated extract of a plant that is kept liquid (that is, no beeswax or oil is added), usually prepared with rubbing alcohol or witch hazel. It is meant to be applied with a cotton ball or cloth. Liniments often include herbs or volatile oils that are sharply fragrant or warming to the skin and are used to reduce muscle aches.

lunar medicine making: I like to steep my tinctures on a new moon and decant them on a full moon (two weeks), or steep them on the full moon and decant them on the following full moon (four weeks). See the sidebar "By the Moon" in chapter 4: Medicine-Making Methods for information on lunar effects on human and botanical systems.

marc: The leftover herbal matter from tincture or oil making; useful for compost.

menstruum: The liquid that will become a tincture. It pulls from the herb all the necessary chemical components and leaves behind cellulose, or indigestible fiber. This liquid makes for a potent, ready-to-assimilate medicine. For a fresh-herb alcohol tincture, the menstruum is 100 percent grain alcohol (190 proof). For a dried-herb alcohol tincture, more water is acceptable, and 40 proof or 50 proof vodkas are fine.

nervine: A class of herbs that soothes, tones, and nourishes the nervous system. These herbs (some sedative, some not) are prized for helping maintain calm and for strengthening the body's response to stress and anxiety.

oil: Liquid pressed from the fruit of a variety of trees and smaller plants. Oils range from clear and tasteless to brightly colored and flavorful. For the purposes of medicine making, oils should be fresh—not stale or rancid—and pharmaceutical or cosmetic grade. For making body oils, use grapeseed, jojoba, sunflower, safflower, hemp, and other stable base oils. For making salves, use thicker oils such as canola and olive. Oil preparations have shelf lives of approximately six to twelve months.

ointment: *See* salve.

plaster: Usually referring to a mustard preparation, a medicinal topical application of warm, wet, ground or dried herbs. This application often covers a wound with a warm, solid barrier as the herbs dry and harden. It is useful as a penetrating cover when made with mustard, which can relieve muscle soreness.

poultice: The medicinal topical application of warm, wet herbs. The herbs are chopped, simmered, and applied directly to the wound. *See also* compress.

powder: The ground form of dried herbal matter; used on the body to remove excess moisture and cool off. Also taken internally in capsule form or stirred into honey.

proof: If you're using 80 proof vodka, this automatically includes a certain percentage of water. For instance, 80 proof means there is 40 percent alcohol and 60 percent water in the bottle. The "proof" is always double the percentage of the alcohol. A bottle of 90 proof vodka contains 45 percent alcohol and 45 percent water. This is an ideal combination. A bottle of 180 proof vodka is straight alcohol and should be mixed with equal parts of water, since many plants release their phytochemicals into only one liquid or the other. For this reason, we combine alcohol and water when making tinctures.

salve: Historically there may have been some difference between salves and ointments, but for the purposes of this book, they are the same. A salve is a blend of oils, herbal extracts, and a solid such as beeswax or petroleum used for topical application to wounds or dry skin. Many commercial ointments contain petroleum-derived base ingredients. Our ancestors used other solids such as beeswax, lard, or lanolin (derived from sheep wool). Beeswax salves make excellent applications for skin, because they create a moisture barrier to keep in skin-healing moisture.

shelf life: The expected length of time a medicinal preparation will be useful.

steep: To brew in hot water. For infusions and decoctions, the water should be brought just to the boil and then poured onto the plant material. Steeping usually lasts from several minutes to several hours or overnight. For tinctures and oils, the water and herbs are allowed to sit at room temperature for the desired length of time (usually two to four weeks).

syrup: A blend of an herbal infusion and a sweetener such as honey, glycerin, or sugar; it is concentrated, sweet, and useful for a variety of medicines and preparations.

tea: A refreshing beverage made from the leaves of *Camellia sinensis*, the tea plant. Tea is the basis for many rich and fragrant drinks, including chai, English Breakfast tea, Irish Breakfast tea, green teas, and white teas. It is naturally caffeinated. *See also* infusion.

tincture: A concentrated herbal application based on the extraction of herbal constituents into a liquid (menstruum). Meant to be taken orally by the drop or teaspoonful. Usually made with grain alcohol such as brandy or vodka, a tincture can also have a vegetable glycerin or vinegar base (with additional water as necessary).

tisane: An herbal beverage. Lighter than tea and usually decaffeinated, tisanes are generally steeped for a short time (5 to 8 minutes) as opposed to infusions and decoctions, which are steeped for several hours.

tonic: A medicinal preparation (as an infusion or sometimes a tincture) that is meant to be taken over a long period of time to nourish and sustain the body. Tonic herbs are safe and nutritious; Ayurvedic tonic herbs are often valued for restoring and rejuvenating the body after an illness.

vegetable glycerin: A sweet-tasting, colorless, and odorless liquid, glycerin is a by-product of both soap making and the biodiesel industry. As sweet as sugar, it does not raise blood sugar levels, and it makes a wonderfully thick, sweet addition to cordials. Many of the recipes in this book call for a simple sugar syrup (a cup water and a cup sugar), but half of this can be substituted with vegetable glycerin if desired. Glycerin is also a valuable menstruum for tinctures; a tincture made with glycerin is called a glycerite. Glycerin is not an acceptable menstruum for tannic acids (plants that contain tannins such as oak, cranesbill, geum, alum root, black alder, sumac, spirea, raspberry leaf, and hemlock tree bark).

Resources

The following list of resources is only a short example of the many exemplary herbal medicine manufacturers, suppliers, and vendors available. But this list is a great start for the beginning herbal medicine crafter and represents what I consider to be among the best in the industry. I've also listed my own business, Vineyard Herbs, as I provide not only ready-made herbal medicines based on the formulas in this book, but also raw materials and supplies that make home crafting easy, affordable, and satisfying.

HERBAL MEDICINE MAKERS AND SUPPLIERS

Vineyard Herbs Teas & Apothecary
www.VineyardHerbs.com; holly@vineyardherbs.com

Supplies hand-harvested wild/organic and hand-crafted herbal simple and compound tinctures, salves, oils, powders, bath salts, liniments, syrups and herbals, and black and green teas. Also supplies crafting kits and supplies. See the website's Workshops page to register for seasonal workshops on Martha's Vineyard, to attend a lecture or conference, or to learn about women's holistic coaching.

Herbalist and Alchemist
www.herbalist-alchemist.com

Run by renowned Western, Eastern, and Cherokee herbalist David Winston. Offers original formulas, simple and compound tinctures, clinical information, and books.

Eclectic Institute
www.eclecticherb.com

Supplies strong herbal tinctures. Established by naturopathic physicians and pharmacists in 1982.

Woodland Essence
www.woodlandessence.com

Offers flower essences from the heart of the northeastern forest, crafted by Kate Gilday.

Mountain Rose Herbs
www.mountainroseherbs.com

Supplies containers, organic bulk raw ingredients, and ready-made herbal medicines.

Sage Mountain Herbs
www.sagemountain.com

Is a resource for herbal education, travel, producers, suppliers, and formulary. Directed by Rosemary Gladstar.

OTHER SUPPLIERS

Glory Bee Foods, Inc.
www.glorybee.com

Honey and bee-related products, beeswax, natural foods, and craft supplies.

Dandy Blend
www.dandyblend.com

Delicious, nourishing coffee substitute. A family-operated company.

Dr. Tieraona Low Dog
www.drlowdog.com

Expert integrative herbalist and medical doctor; women's health issues; and ADD/ADHD solutions.

EDUCATIONAL PROGRAMS

Heritage & Healing Herbal Studies Program
www.VineyardHerbs.com

Designed for beginning and advanced herbalists, life and wellness coaches, and alternative healing arts professionals, this home study course offers an inspiring educational opportunity to study the botany, chemistry, heritage, and folklore of herbal medicine from author, speaker, and herbalist Holly Bellebuono. Learn in a supportive environment with personal attention, receiving detailed instruction in herbal identification, harvesting, processing, and application for family or professional use. Also discover the broader context of community herbalism, women's health, historical and global pharmacy, and the heritage of the world's healing traditions. The course is provided in written form with supplementary audio CD recordings, with a completion certificate awarded and retreat opportunities for continuing herbal studies. Email holly@vineyardherbs.com or call (508) 687-9600 for complete details and to register.

CONFERENCES AND ASSOCIATIONS

New England Women's Herbal Conference
www.womensherbalconference.com

Carefree, lovely, wild, and exuberant. This women-only conference is a wonderful gathering of creative spirits celebrating the bounty of herbs.

International Herb Symposium
www.internationalherbsymposium.com

More academic and useful for herbalists who wish to learn more in-depth information about herbal medicine, as well as doctors, nurses, midwives, and other healers who wish to gain a solid perspective on botanical integration.

Breitenbush Herbal Conference
breitensbushherbalconference.com

Held on the West Coast, a gathering for sharing, exchanging, learning, and growing.

United Plant Savers
www.unitedplantsavers.org

A nonprofit dedicated to protecting native medicinal plants and their habitats.

Traditional Healers Exchange and Advancement (THEA) International
www.VineyardHerbs.com

A nonprofit planned for the sole purpose of bringing healers and students together to advance the sharing of traditional knowledge. Provides scholarships for learning and stipends for teaching.

Green Nations Gathering
www.greennationsgathering.com

A vibrant community of plant lovers from around the world that comes together to celebrate the beauty and bounty of plants.

Northeast Herbal Association
www.northeastherbal.org

"Dedicated to merging the ancient traditions of Herbalism with the needs and development of the modern-day Herbalist."

American Botanical Council
www.herbalgram.org

Advises the media and the public on emerging herbal science.

American Herb Association
www.ahaherb.com

Promotes the understanding and ecological use of medicinal herbs and aromatherapy.

Suggested Reading and References

I've enjoyed a wonderful hobby throughout the years: collecting herbals from around the world. There are many useful botanical and healing books, and the ones listed here are those I turn to again and again. I highly recommend them for instruction in herbal medicine, gardening, cooking, health care, women's issues, and modern/traditional herbalism.

Buhner, Stephen Harrod. *Healing Lyme: Natural Healing and Prevention of Lyme Borreliosis and Its Coinfections*. Randolph, Vt.: Raven Press, 2005.

The last word on Lyme disease, its prevention and cure, with all the scientific oomph of the laboratory community. Very scientifically written, it takes focus to follow.

Cowan, Eliot. *Plant Spirit Medicine: Healing with the Power of Plants*. Columbus, N.C.: Swan Raven and Co., 1995.

A revolutionary book that teaches the plant world is intelligent, spiritual, and completely connected to our own.

David, Laurie, and Kirstin Uhrenholdt. *The Family Dinner: Great Ways to Connect with Your Kids, One Meal at a Time*. New York, N.Y.: Grand Central Life & Style, 2010.

Use this warm-hearted book as an idea generator for wonderful ways to spend dinnertime with your family. It's full of delicious and whole-food based recipes, tips, games, and photos.

de Bairacli Levy, Juliette. *Herbal Handbook for Everyone*. London: Faber and Faber, 1966.

Valuable and authoritative. This and other books by the same author have been reproduced and are available through Ash Tree Publishing (www.ashtreepublishing.com).

Juliette de Bairacli Levy was a veterinary holistic healer whose successful remedies form the basis for many herbalists today.

Gibbons, Euell. *Stalking the Healthful Herbs*. New York, N.Y.: David McKay Co. Inc., 1966.

I dote on Euell Gibbons as if he were an uncle. I never met him but feel, through reading his charming and down-to-earth books, as if I've walked around in the woods with him, chewing wild mint.

Gibbons, Euell. *Stalking the Wild Asparagus*. New York, N.Y.: David McKay Co. Inc., 1962.

This book, together with *Stalking the Healthful Herbs*, recounts Euell's adventures finding, harvesting, cooking, and eating dozens of wild plants.

Gladstar, Rosemary. *Herbal Healing for Women: Simple Home Remedies for Women of All Ages*. New York, N.Y.: Fireside/Simon and Schuster, 1993.

Rosemary is the cornerstone of the American herbalist movement, an ambassador for the plant world, and a persuasive teacher. Her books are personal and lovely.

Gladstar, Rosemary. *Rosemary Gladstar's Family Herbal: A Guide to Living Life with Energy, Health and Vitality*. North Adams, Mass.: Storey Publishing, 2001.

Filled with lovely antiqued photographs, Rosemary's book is a beautiful collection of recipes, insights, and ideas.

Green, James. *The Herbal Medicine-Maker's Handbook: A Home Manual*. Berkeley, Calif.: Crossing Press, 2000.

James Green lists step-by-step processes for making both simple and complex herbal remedies for the home herbalist and for the professional formulator. Use these guidelines as a benchmark for experimenting with your own herbal medicines.

Griggs, Barbara. *Green Pharmacy: The History and Evolution of Western Herbal Medicine*. Rochester, Vt.: Healing Arts Press, 1997.

An encyclopedic study of herbal medicine from Galen and Paracelsus to the Regulars of Twentieth Century America. Excellent resource for dates, people, doctors, events, discoveries, inventions, fights, heroes, and disasters of medicine.

Hoffmann, David. *The Herbal Handbook*. Rochester, Vt.: Healing Arts Press, 1988.

I earned a certificate in phytotherapy from David and have collected many of his books. His focus is on the chemical benefits inherent in botany as well as the holistic framework in which we practice herbal healing.

Jordan, Michael. *The Green Mantle: An Investigation into Our Lost Knowledge of Plants*. London: Cassell and Co, 1991.

Mythology, especially the lure, lore, and love of plants. Explores the intercultural religions of "vegetative" gods and goddesses.

Mabey, Richard. *The New Age Herbalist: How to Use Herbs for Healing, Nutrition, Body Care, and Relaxation*. New York, N.Y.: Collier/Macmillian Publishing, 1988.

Thorough, with illustrations and photographs. Topics organized by plant and pathology.

Návar, Maria Margarita. *Zapotec Woman of the Clouds: The Life of Enriqueta Contreras Contreras*. Austin, Tex.: Zapotec Press, 2010.

I was blessed to meet both Margie Návar and Doña Enriqueta Contreras while completing my documentary of global traditional healing practitioners. Margie's book is a rare and beautiful celebration of traditional healing, especially of the life of one extremely influential healer and midwife. Written in both Spanish and English, with lovely full-color photographs of Doña Enriqueta and Oaxaca, Mexico, this is a powerful tribute to a dynamic woman's devotion to midwifery and her contribution to an incredible heritage.

Tompkins, Peter, and Christopher Bird. *The Secret Life of Plants*. New York, N.Y.: Harper & Row Publishers, 1973.

A rather esoteric yet thoroughly fascinating study of people's attempts to understand the physical, spiritual, and energetic nature of plants.

Vargas, Pattie, and Rich Gulling. *Cordials from Your Kitchen: Easy, Elegant Liqueurs You Can Make and Give*. North Adams, Mass.: Storey Publishing, 1997.

Easy-to-follow recipes that are easy to alter; lots of ideas.

Weed, Susun. *Healing Wise* (Wise Woman Herbal Series). Woodstock, N.Y.: Ash Tree Publishing, 1989.

A lovely and in-depth look at six common herbs; a fascinating way to listen to their teachings and learn to use them.

Index

About the Author

HOLLY BELLEBUONO, M.P.A., C.H., C.P.C., is a respected writer, motivational speaker, and women's holistic coach, offering one-on-one women's empowerment programs that nourish the body, mind, and spirit through connecting with plants. Holly also instructs the distance-learning course Heritage & Healing Herbal Studies Program, a custom educational curriculum designed to inspire and educate the family herbalist, wellness coach, and healing arts professional. With seventeen years experience harvesting, formulating, and educating about herbal medicine, Holly is president and C.V.O of Vineyard Herbs Teas & Apothecary, a full-service, award-winning holistic retailer providing original herbal formulas for organic markets and boutiques. She is a feature writer for magazines, and her slide documentary and lecture *Healing Across 6 Continents* teaches the inherent value of the world's vast healing traditions. A native of Asheville, North Carolina, Holly can often be found hiking or gardening at her home on Martha's Vineyard with her husband and two children.

The following recipes are trademarks of Vineyard Herbs Teas & Apothecary: Vineyard Herbs Breast Milk Fountain, Breast Milk Fountain Tea, Children's Sleepytime Tonic, Katama Chamomile Calming Blend Tea, Wild Yam PMS Jam, Menopause Friend Tincture, Martha's Vineyard Wise Woman Herbal Tea, Women's Ultimate Tonic Elixir, Squibnocket Soother, Chilmark Chai, West Chop Winter Tea for Colds and Flu, Elderberry-Ginger Syrup for Colds and Flu, Rosemary's Blessing First Aid Ointment, Bye-Bye Bugs Insect Repellent Spray, Digestive Aid/Gas Relief Tincture, Menemsha Mint Tea, Aquinnah Cliffs Licorice Tea, Mood Mend Tincture, Vineyard Summer Lemon Tea, and Edgartown English Breakfast.

Designed by Lora Zorian

Library of Congress Cataloging-in-Publication Data

Bellebuono, Holly.
The essential herbal for natural health: how to transform
easy-to-find herbs into healing remedies for the whole family
/ Holly Bellebuono.
p. cm.
ISBN 978-1-59030-947-6 (pbk.)
1. Naturopathy. 2. Herbs—Therapeutic use. 3. Self-care, Health.
4. Alternative medicine. I. Title.
RZ440.B45 2012
615'.321—dc23
2011022507